THE DOCTOR IN THE
MIRROR

LIVING A LONGER, HEALTHIER,
MORE JOYFUL LIFE STARTS WITH <u>YOU</u>.

REED V. TUCKSON, MD

United HealthCare Services, Inc.

Hardcover
ISBN-13: 978-0-98476-220-0

Library of Congress Catalog Number: 2011941629

Printed in Canada

First Printing: January 2012

16 15 14 13 12   5 4 3 2 1

_____

United HealthCare Services, Inc.

www.doctorinthemirror.com

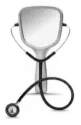

To the nearly 100 million Americans who are over 50, some of whom are struggling against great odds to live healthy and fulfilling lives. And to health professionals of every discipline whose personal mission is to help each of us promote our health, prevent disease, and restore our maximum function. Finally, to my wife, my mother, and my brother, each of whom in their own way inspire me to serve the health needs of others.

TABLE OF CONTENTS

SECTION 1: LIFESTYLE

SECTION 2: MEDICAL DECISIONS

SECTION 3: HOME AND FAMILY

ACKNOWLEDGMENTS

There are many who journeyed alongside me in the creation of this book. Kerry Casey, my editor, colleague, and confidante. Terry Clark for his inspiring vision. My outstanding physician colleagues for their inexhaustible collaboration and clinical expertise. The hundreds of care managers I'm privileged to work with at UnitedHealthcare, whose experience, insight, and compassion are unmatched. The entire Periscope team for their extraordinary creativity and expertise. The dedicated group at Soulo Communications. And finally, Jane Devine and Jane Pennington, whose unwavering support—and countless gentle prods—helped make it possible that I write this book and complete its many related activities without losing my sense of humor.

INTRODUCTION

*"Tell a person to get healthy, and he or she will walk away.
Teach a person to get healthy, and he or she
will take a brisk walk with you."*

—Dr. Reed Tuckson

✚ MEET DR. YOU

Would you like to know one of the most often-overlooked medical truths? No one knows what's going on inside your body like you do. And no one knows what's on your mind like you do, either. So, given the proper assistance, who do you think is eminently qualified to be one of your key health advisors? Just look in the mirror. You'll be face-to-face with one of the most capable doctors you've ever met. You'll be looking at the amazing, the brilliant, the esteemed Dr. You.

If you think about it, Dr. You has been seeing you for your whole life. Now, of course, we all need to visit physicians like myself, and specialists, and other health professionals to help prevent and treat disease on your life journey—and the health system will be there for you. My point is this: so much of *your* wellness is in *your* hands. Dr. You is a specialist who can work alongside your other doctors to make you as strong, healthy, and full of life as can be.

My goal in this book is to teach, not tell. We've all been told for years, "You need to do this" or "Why don't you do that?" Instead, we'll dig into the everyday barriers between you and better health, and you'll learn how to pull them down, brick by brick.

Today's the day you recognize that you are the doctor in the mirror, and that you truly can become the strongest advocate for your health. Not overnight, but over time. By opening this book, and being equally open to its content, you will have the information and strategies, the ideas and resources to improve and extend your life.

In medicine, there is something called the doctor-patient relationship. It's a concept centered on honesty, dignity, and trust. In this book, I want to introduce the concept of the author-reader relationship. It's centered on those same qualities so we can form a relationship through these pages—built on an open, trusting conversation. That's how barriers come down, not only between us, but between you and your best possible health.

I'm not big on complicated doctor-speak or aloof professionalism. I hope you'll find the following pages to be an engaging, common sense guide to everyday health issues. Some of the things I'll share with you, you may have heard before. What's different, however, is we will talk about the barriers keeping you from your goals, and ways to overcome them.

This book has been divided into three main sections. Each section digs deeply into the areas that affect you most as you age: your lifestyle, your medical needs, and your home and family.

"In many ways, this book is like your medical residency. It will teach Dr. You what you need to know to take better care of yourself—and what could be more important than that?"

I like to say I'm a 60-something doctor with 40-something years of experience. Chances are, you know the importance of experience and perspective when it comes to dispensing advice because you have plenty of wisdom yourself.

My career has taken me all over this wonderful country, and it still does today. As an MD, I've gathered knowledge one case, one patient at a time. As a former Commissioner of Health, I've learned about grassroots medical challenges confronting American families and communities. And now, as the Chief of Medical Affairs at UnitedHealth Group, one of the nation's

preeminent health care insurers, I have a national view of
health issues gleaned from serving more than 70 million people.

This diversity of experience helps me understand today's
critical health challenges, and the best practices to prevent
and remedy those challenges. Over my life in medicine, I have
come to embrace the idea that health is not the absence of pain
or disease. Rather, health is the mental, physical, and spiritual
well-being of a person. With that definition in mind we will
pursue health, and in doing so, your life can be improved and
extended.

In many ways, this book is like your medical residency. It
will teach Dr. You what you need to know to take better care
of yourself—and what could be more important than that? So
read on and live well. And in the end, follow the doctor's orders,
because the doctor is you.

SECTION 1
LIFESTYLE

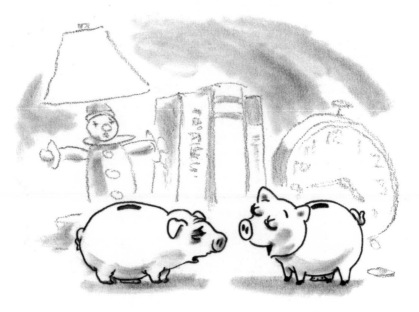

*"You look like a million bucks.
How'd ya do it?"*

"One penny at a time."

You are your lifestyle; it's a simple truth. Take a quick inventory
of how you live: your behaviors, attitudes, and habits. Guess
what you'll discover? Essentially, how you live is how you feel.
If you don't feel as well as you'd like, it's time to make some
lifestyle changes.

So, how do you improve the health of your lifestyle? Start by looking in the mirror. Who are you? What person do you see? What health issues do you bring to the looking glass? Okay, that's you, past and present. But this book is about the future you. What do you want to do with the rest of your life? What barriers are holding you back? What are your goals?

For me, as a cyclist, there are a few steep hills on my training rides that I want to climb as fast as the young studs. For you, your goal may be larger than that. I just read about a 61-year-old woman who set out to swim from Cuba to Florida (without a shark cage!). Or maybe your goal is more modest, like walking three mornings per week with a friend.

The point is: the size of the goal doesn't matter, it's *having* goals that matters—that's how you make healthy progress. We're not looking to change lifestyles overnight, we're looking to change them over time. As the doctor in the mirror, what would you advise yourself to do?

One aspect of my career that I really enjoy is meeting people: ordinary folks to true geniuses. We eventually get talking about health and they say things like, "Dr, Reed, my lifestyle is pretty good, but my health is lousy. I think I got stuck with bad genes." Or "I've been surrounded by unhealthy behavior my whole life, so what can I do about it now?" Or "The way I live, I can't believe I'm not sicker than I am."

No matter how different the people and their stories are, one thing stays the same: their lifestyles have more to do with their health than any other factor.

So, dear Reader, let's begin by looking at the broader national lifestyle, and see how culture affects your health—and boy does it ever! We'll look at disease, and how to prevent it. Then you can have a look in the mirror, where Dr. You can put together a simple, personal lifestyle plan that promotes health. Let's call it a lifestyle re-style.

CHAPTERS IN THIS SECTION:

1. Health in America

2. Bad Habits

3. Diet

4. Be Active

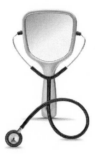

CHAPTER 1

HEALTH IN AMERICA

✚ THE SLIPPERY SLOPE OF POOR HEALTH

America is the greatest country on earth, but when it comes to health, America isn't doing so well. And like it or not, national trends do trickle down (or crash down) on us as individuals. So it's very important that you're aware of how our country's health is trending. I'm here to tell you it's not trending the way any of us would like.

First off, America is not number one. Not in health, that is. It appears we're on a slippery slope moving in the wrong

direction. Since the year 2000, our progress in improving overall healthiness has slowed. Case in point: guess how many
countries have life expectancies that exceed ours in the United
States? Five? Twenty? Fifty? If you said 50 you'd be darn close.
Forty-nine countries have higher life expectancy rates than
America.[1] Have a look at the list provided. I have a hunch
you'll be surprised by many of the countries that beat America
in the life expectancy department.

LIFE EXPECTANCY AT BIRTH

RANK	COUNTRY	YEARS
1	Monaco	89.73
2	Macau	84.41
3	San Marino	83.01
4	Andorra	82.43
5	Japan	82.25
6	Guernsey	82.16
7	Singapore	82.14
8	Hong Kong	82.04
9	Australia	81.81
10	Italy	81.77
49	Portugal	78.54
50	**UNITED STATES**	**78.37**
51	Taiwan	78.32

Here are a few implications. Let's say you're going to be
a new grandparent. Forty countries have lower—as in better—infant mortality rates (death in the first year of life) than

DR. YOU MEDICAL NOTE:

A Japanese granddaughter is expected to outlive an American granddaughter by six years.

we do.[2] And further, let's say you're blessed with a beautiful granddaughter. Statistically, broken down by gender, she will have 81 years to pursue her dreams in the U.S. compared to 87 years in Japan.[3] Six more years were she not born in America. That's a big deal! And it's unacceptable.

So how else does our nation's suboptimal health affect you? Tragically, your risk of being afflicted by multiple chronic illnesses is on the rise. That translates to far too many premature deaths for senior Americans. When a life is cut short, you and your loved ones are robbed of precious time together.

Dear Reader, we must get off this slippery slope of declining health. The effects are too dangerous to ignore. I know that this country can do better—starting with you. And I'm going to show you how in simple, practical ways.

✚ BOY OH BOY IS AMERICA BOOMING

Here's a number that's sure to be a showstopper at your next backyard get-together: Baby Boomers, those born in the birth explosion from 1946 to 1964, are turning 65 at a rate of roughly 9000 a day.[4] Or try this: well over 200,000 Americans turn 65 each month.[5] That's mind-boggling.

> **"A mind-boggling 200,000 Americans turn 65 each month."**

To get a sense of the scope of that number, Google "Michigan Stadium in Ann Arbor." It's a gigantic stadium, holding roughly 107,000 fans, one of the largest capacities in college football. Now double that crowd and that's about how many folks will turn 65—this month! And next month, and the next, and the next.

What this means is we're in uncharted waters when it comes to the number of older Americans alive today. We're learning how to meet the health demands of our aging population as we go. As a physician friend of mine likes to say, we're building the airplane as we fly.

I'll give you one last example, and this one, once you've had time to digest it, will blow you away: approximately two-thirds of all the people in the history of the world who have ever lived past age 65 are alive today.[6] Amazing! But as we will continue to review in this section, it's not just aging that presents problems for us as individuals or as a nation, it's also that we're experiencing worrisome increases in preventable chronic illness.

So, you may be thinking, what do all these numbers really mean? They mean that health professionals, hospitals, nursing

DR. YOU MEDICAL NOTE:

Approximately two-thirds of all the people in the history of the world who have ever lived past age 65 are alive today!

homes, the health care financing system, and essential community-based service organizations are all facing challenges that they've never seen before. We have no proven playbook for what we're facing. So, like America has always done, we all need to step up, meet the health care challenge, and do our part to help lessen the strain.

✚ WHAT IS "NORMAL AGING"?

No one is especially fond of aging. But, as I like to say, there's no future in the alternative. So, as you age, what changes should you expect?

Throughout this book, we'll delve into more and more specifics, but for now, I'd like you to think about your health's "big picture." As we age, we change. Sometimes the changes are for the better, sometimes the changes are normal, sometimes our changing bodies are reason for concern. You need to recognize and know the differences.

A few of the changes for the better as we age are increased wisdom, patience, judgment, and perspective.

Some of the changes for the worse we'll cover shortly.

Let's talk now about noticeable changes that are expected and normal. (However, that doesn't mean that there's nothing you can do about them.) Here's where Dr. You steps in to observe your aging, and gains a few tips and strategies on what to do about these normal occurrences.

Skin. Yes, there will be wrinkles, despite what the "age-defying" advertisements promise. What happens is that your oil glands will start producing less oil, leading to drier skin, and sometimes itchier and more irritated skin. So it's time to be on the lookout for dry skin, and to become a regular user of moisturizer. (Yes, guys, us too.) Sunscreen and UV-protective clothing are absolutely essential to protect you from sunburn, "liver spots," and skin cancer. The sun is your friend, but only on your terms. See the Centers for Disease Control and Prevention's skin cancer prevention page for more: www.cdc.gov/cancer/skin/basic_info/prevention.html.

Eyesight. Your vision won't be as sharp, and additionally you'll lose some peripheral vision and depth perception. While driving, glare and night vision will become increasingly challenging. Plan accordingly with proper sunglasses and daytime driving to avoid rush hour whenever possible. And don't forget your yearly eye exam; it's the best way to identify and treat eye problems early.

Hearing. Higher-frequency sounds like the little voices of grandchildren will become increasingly difficult to hear. Many times, hearing difficulty is a simple case of earwax buildup, so have your ears checked. While you're at it, get your hearing tested, and if need be, purchase hearing aids rather than continuing to turn up the television or use your spouse as a hearing aid. ("What did he say?") There are a number of very lightweight, very discreet hearing products that can greatly improve the quality of your life—and your safety. Hearing loss puts untold strain on relationships, and is linked with depression. Please, have your hearing tested annually.

Bones. Your bones will become less dense as you age because calcium and phosphate, the two minerals that are essential for normal bone formation, are reabsorbed out of your bones and then out of your body. This can lead to osteoporosis. Weight-bearing exercise such as walking, and weight-resistance exercises with light hand weights or stretchy bands become more and more important to keeping healthy bones healthy with every additional year. In an upcoming chapter we'll discuss some great, simple physical activities to keep your bones, muscles, and heart strong. Also talk to your doctor about calcium and vitamin D supplements to help preserve bone mass and prevent hip fractures.

Musculature. Normal aging results in measurable loss of muscle mass and strength. What's important is that you take the necessary steps to limit the loss. You can't make muscle as fast as you once could, but no doubt about it, you can still make muscle. Don't accept weak arms as a mandate of normal aging. I'm going to suggest some easy-to-do exercises in chapter four, but if you're raring to go right now, see www.easyforyou.info. It's a wonderful introductory exercise website.

Metabolism. Metabolism is both the rate at which you burn calories and how the nutrients from those calories are used to maintain a healthy body. For most, as you age, your metabolism slows. That's normal. What that means is it takes longer to burn off the same size slice of cake on your fifty-fifth birthday than it did on your twentieth. (Maybe you should run around the cake to blow out the candles?) Here's the good news: exercise and maintaining or building muscle mass can keep your metabolism really humming along. Remember, your metabolism loves muscle. Thanks to muscle, your body is better at burning calories—even when you're not exercising. Now that's what I call having your cake and eating it, too.

Brain. Because of breakthroughs in imaging technology, we are learning more and more about the brain every day. Nonetheless, much about this most vital organ is still a mystery, especially with regard to aging. There is one thing, though, we know for certain. It's normal to expect some short-term memory issues (senior moments) such as, "Where the heck did I park?" But it's important to note that a pattern of increased frequency of memory loss, or memory loss of familiar things like the name of a family member or your home address is NOT normal. There is a simple point of agreement among neurologists that I'll translate into everyday English: use it or lose it! Many experts agree that cognitive challenges—keeping the mind active—can "turn on" neurons and create new ones in the adult brain. So don't just veg out in front of the TV. Get into the habit of reading regularly as well as doing Sudoku and crossword puzzles, too. You can find great brainteasers on the Internet, and they're free.

"Your brain: use it or lose it."

Heart. Your heart is amazing. Approximately the size of your clenched fist, an average healthy adult heart weighs about 12 ounces (roughly the weight of this book). And what a hard worker! The circulatory system that your heart services is no small network. Stretched end-to-end, the arteries, veins, and other vessels would span about 60,000 miles. Considering that the United States is about 3,000 miles coast to coast, that's 20 cross-country trips that one heroic little pump is responsible for.[7] The aging heart can't pump as strongly as a 20-year-old heart because it becomes less efficient and larger with age. That said, a healthy heart will pump valiantly for up to 100-plus years if you treat it well. Put your hand on your chest. Feel it beat? That's YOUR life there. Now with your hand to your

WHAT A PUMP!

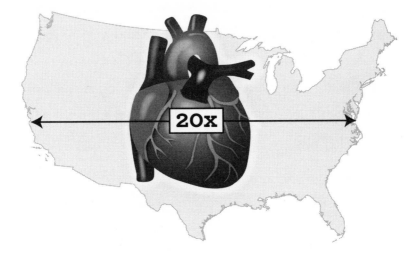

Your heart pumps blood through a circulatory system that if stretched end-to-end, would span about 60,000 miles—that's 20 cross-country trips. Keep it healthy.

heart, vow to be a good Dr. You and take better care of your heart. The following pages will show you how.

With aging comes inevitable change. By age 80, for example, expect to be two inches shorter than you were at 30. But there are many health issues you can and should actively work on rather than writing them off as inevitable. Let's work on what we can control, because it's a long and exciting list. As for those two inches you'll lose in height, don't sweat it. You're not getting two inches shorter; you're just becoming more down-to-earth, right?

✛ THIS IS NOT NORMAL AGING

You've probably heard it said, or maybe said it yourself, "Ah, what's the big deal? That's just what happens when you get old." Well just a darn minute. Says who?

As we've talked about since page one of this book, the doctor in the mirror is <u>you</u>. You have the best sense of what's normal when it comes to your body and what's going on inside. Call it a "gut feeling."

"You're not getting shorter as you age; you're just becoming more down-to-earth, right?"

When you notice a change that doesn't seem normal, please, you need to identify it EARLY and go see your doctor. When conditions are caught early, we can focus on the necessary preventive treatments as you work closely with your health care team, as well as dealing with this issue yourself and with your family.

Let's begin by clearing the air of some popular misinformation by briefly reviewing what is NOT normal aging. This way, Dr. You will have a baseline of medical information, along with your gut instinct, by which to make better health decisions.

✚ MEMORY LOSS AND DEMENTIA

Dementia is a syndrome of several conditions that results in the progressive and permanent loss of brain function. It affects normal activities and social relationships. Dementia can show up in problems such as forgetting the names of family members, getting lost on familiar routes, or repeatedly misplacing things. Other symptoms include personality changes, poor decision-making ability, and the loss of social skills. It's important to see your doctor if these symptoms persist, and identify treatable conditions early. For conditions such as Alzheimer's disease, for which scientists continue to work on effective treatments, early identification can allow for planning and the minimization of their impact until better treatments become available. There is evidence that some forms of physical and mental exercise can help slow down dementia. But you, your doctor, and your loved ones need to team up and make a plan. Here are two good sources for more information: the Alzheimer's Association, www.alz.org, and the National Institute on Aging: Alzheimer's Disease Education & Referral Center, www.nia.nih.gov/alzheimers.

❝Depression is not a sign of weakness. And it's certainly not something you have to live with.❞

+ DEPRESSION

Sadness, helplessness, and hopelessness. If these three words apply to your mood for more than two weeks, you need to talk to a nurse or doctor. Be honest with yourself. This is important. Depression is not to be underestimated for many reasons, least of all because depression and physical health are interrelated: one can worsen the other. There are many non-habit-forming medications that can be taken effectively for a limited time (often a year or less) causing few or no side effects. There are also non-drug options like talk therapy and exercise.

Depression is not a sign of weakness, and many times it's not just a dark cloud that will pass on its own. And it's certainly not something you have to live with. A good source for more information can be found at the National Institute of Mental Health, www.nimh.nih.gov.

+ INCONTINENCE

Incontinence, or the loss of control of urine or bowel movements, is a sign of an underlying problem. It could be caused by a number of things, including infection, adverse reaction to medication, and even, ironically, constipation. Many treatments have been successful in overcoming incontinence, including behavioral techniques (exercises), medication, and surgery. Remember, there are many good options for dealing with incontinence. Ignoring or hiding it is not one of them. Here is a good source for more information: the National Institute on Aging: www.nia.nih.gov/HealthInformation/Publications/urinary.html.

✛ ANEMIA

Anemia is a condition in which you lack enough healthy red blood cells to carry vital oxygen to your tissues. If you feel exhausted, dizzy, weak, short of breath, if your skin is pale, your hands and feet are cold, or your balance is poor, these are often telltale signs. There are many types of anemia, and a simple blood test is the starting point for finding the correct treatment. It's important to find the cause early, as anemia may be a warning sign of a more serious illness. Dramatic improvements in your energy, vitality, and strength can often be made with dietary changes and supplements. A good source for more information can be found by visiting www.healthinaging.org then type "anemia" into the search bar.

✛ DISINTEREST IN SEX

It's almost impossible to watch a sporting event or a prime-time drama these days without seeing a commercial of a 60-something stud with a potent sex pill tucked into the pocket of his snug-fitting jeans, climbing onto a motorcycle, and riding

> **DR. YOU MEDICAL NOTE:**
>
> Sometimes pain screams. Sometimes pain speaks to you in a low, constant, nagging voice. What pain is saying is, "Hey, this isn't normal. Have me checked out."

off into the sunset with his significant other's arms wrapped around his waist. Hmm, reality check? But allow me one small plug for these "passionate" commercials: they bring the once-taboo issue of low to abnormal sexual activity into the public conversation (although the living room with your granddaughter might not be the ideal place for such a conversation). My point is that sexual disinterest and impotence affects millions of seniors and it should be addressed openly and honestly with Dr. You, your physician, and your partner. It could be related to a medical condition, but there are a number of treatments that your doctor can privately talk you and your partner through. And no, not all solutions require a motorcycle.

✚ PAIN

In America, we pride ourselves on toughness. It must have been all those westerns we watched growing up. You remember the scene: a cowboy has taken a bullet to the shoulder. How does he prepare to have the hunk of lead dug out? All he needs is a few swallows of whiskey and a gun belt to bite down on.

Ha! More realistically, pain is your body telling you something—and that something is not—"ignore me." Sometimes pain screams. Sometimes pain speaks to you in a low, constant, nagging voice. Sometimes pain sits like a weight pressing down on your chest. What pain is saying is, "Hey, this isn't normal. Have me checked out." Once again, it's critical to find the cause before a potentially serious problem becomes a serious problem.

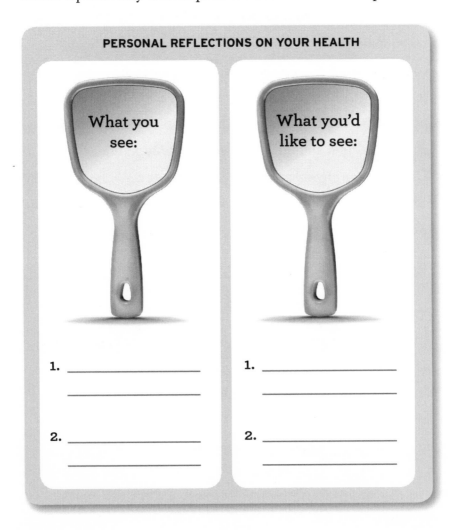

PERSONAL REFLECTIONS ON YOUR HEALTH

What you see:

What you'd like to see:

1. _____

2. _____

1. _____

2. _____

There are treatment options for pain that range from simple to surgical. The key is that life's too short to not have quality. Don't live with pain. Throw it out of the house for being loud and nagging. Start by talking to your primary care physician. Preferably, one who isn't wearing a cowboy hat.

That being said, there are people I meet who are currently overmedicating themselves, and do so regularly—often with over-the-counter pain medication. They seem unwilling to tolerate any discomfort at all and believe in a practice known as "a pill for every ill." Dear Reader, it's all about using your judgment and observing your body closely over time. Like I say, nobody knows you better.

The last point I'd like to make about the conditions we just reviewed is something I call "watch out for the rug." It's a simple way to sum up what we've just covered about abnormal aging and what to do when symptoms arise. When something is wrong, don't dismiss it or "sweep it under the rug" because it will likely get worse with time. Just remember this little saying: if you sweep something under the rug, you're going to trip over it later. Now that's good advice for Dr. You.

✚ THE BIG THREE CHRONIC ILLNESSES

As I mentioned before, not only are we aging as a nation, we're also experiencing soaring increases in chronic illness. The Centers for Disease Control and Prevention report that almost 80%

of Americans aged 55-plus have at least one chronic condition. And nearly 25% of those 65-plus have three or more chronic conditions. This seriously diminishes our quality of life and the security of our finances.

So, in the interest of self-preservation, what "not normal" conditions are the most prevalent? What should you be looking out for, and working hardest to prevent? To put it bluntly, what is making us sickest, what's killing us, and what do we do to avoid it? Let's look at the big ones.

✚ ARTHRITIS

The most common chronic illness for aging adults is arthritis. We've all heard the word, but what is arthritis? In short, it's joint inflammation that restricts movement. And as you instinctively knew from the age you first escaped from your crib and began crawling every which direction, moving is something we need to do to stay healthy. There are many types of arthritis and I'm going to examine every one of them in detail right now. (Remember, joking and good humor are effective, affordable medicines, and will be dispensed throughout these pages.)

THREE WAYS TO FIGHT ARTHRITIS

Movement
Keep excess weight off joints
Simple strength training

Actually, the one nugget of arthritis information I'd like you to take from this book is that many forms of arthritis can be prevented and treated by means *outside* of medication. Does this mean you never take medication for arthritis? No it does not. There are many treatments that are complementary to medication. But as a country, we need to do more to keep arthritis from getting to a point where medication is the only treatment. How? One: keep joints moving. Two: keep excess body weight off joints. Three: start a simple strength training routine. These three decisions will go a long way toward knocking arthritis off the top of the chronic illnesses chart. We, all of us 50-plus, need to commit to them.

Another point: a recent study indicated that people who have arthritis may have fewer days of feeling mentally and physically well, and are more likely to feel unwell.[8] What does this mean? Arthritis affects your mental well-being, too. How can I make that point more strongly? This is not a picture I enjoy painting, but it's effective: arthritis of the joints often leads to arthritis of the soul. Please, don't let that happen.

What if arthritis is in the family? There's no escaping it, right? Wrong. Some forms of arthritis do have genetic links, but that does not mean that you are certain to develop it. And if you do develop arthritis, there are numerous ways to minimize the consequences.

Determination is strong medicine. Action is strong medicine. A support system is strong medicine. In the chapters ahead we'll talk about everything from diet to exercise to creating a family safety net to help in the fight against arthritis and other conditions. A great source for more information is the Arthritis Foundation at www.arthritis.org. I like it because it helps people who have all types of arthritis, and all severities, to maximize their function.

✚ CVD

The biggest concern for seniors today is a big C, but not *the* big C. Care to guess which C I'm referring to? It's cardiovascular disease, also known as CVD. That's the number-one killer for seniors 65-plus.[9]

What is cardiovascular disease, and why should you care? I'll begin with the second part of that question first. You should care because, like I said, it's the leading cause of death among seniors. So, does that mean cardiovascular disease is a death sentence and there's little or nothing we can do about it? Heck no! (I occasionally use more colorful language but I promised my editors I'd behave.) We'll be addressing how you can greatly reduce your chances of getting CVD shortly. But first, let me tell you what it is.

Cardio comes from the Greek *kardia*, which means heart, and vascular is related to blood vessels, arteries, and veins. So a disease affecting the heart and blood vessels is known as cardio-vascular disease.

"Every time you pick up this book, I want you to congratulate yourself because you are taking your health into your own hands."

Many times, CVD is caused by hypertension, or high blood pressure, which we'll talk about in the next chapter. CVD is also associated with atherosclerosis, a condition in which fatty material, called plaque, collects along the walls of arteries. This fatty material will thicken, then harden, forming calcium deposits. This buildup narrows the arteries, making it harder for blood to flow through them. In combination with other factors, it can eventually block arteries, causing a blood clot that can lead to heart attack or stroke.

Think of it this way: your artery is a highway; your blood flow is your car; your heart is your destination. Very early in the morning, just like very early in life, the traffic flow on your highway is amazing. Your car (your blood flow) is zoom-ing right along, getting where it needs to go (your heart) lickety-split.

Later in the day, just as can happen later in life, the high-way slows. Let's say there are stalled cars on either shoulder of

DR. YOU MEDICAL NOTE:

Half of men and one-third of women will develop cancer.

the road—those would be the plaque deposits we talked about. Everything is slowing down, there's congestion, and your car (your blood flow) can only move at a crawl to its destination. Now let's say all this congestion causes an accident in the middle of the highway and all traffic stops. That's a blood clot in your artery, causing a heart attack or stroke.

The key is to keep the highway free of stalled cars in the first place. More times than not, those stalled cars are high-cholesterol vehicles. Fatty, processed foods are typically the culprit. In upcoming chapters, we'll talk about simple things you can do to significantly reduce your chances of CVD—including mastering the reading of food labels and identifying bad fats—so you can keep that traffic flowing freely.

✚ CANCER

Half of men and one-third of women will develop cancer in their lifetime.[10] Cancer is a general name given to over 100 diseases in which cells grow out of control and invade other tissue. Left untreated, this abnormal growth can cause serious illness and even death. In most cases, the cancer cells form a tumor (although not all tumors are cancerous). But with some cancers such as leukemia, tumors rarely form. Instead, these cancer cells circulate in the blood, growing in body tissue. When cancer cells move to other parts of the body and begin to grow and form new tumors, it's called metastasis.

9 MOST COMMON CANCERS

1. Non-melanoma skin cancer
2. Lung cancer
3. Prostate cancer
4. Colon and rectal cancers
5. Bladder cancer
6. Non-Hodgkin's lymphoma
7. Melanoma
8. Kidney (Renal Cell) cancer
9. Leukemia

4 WAYS TO REDUCE YOUR RISK

1. Monitor sun exposure and protect your skin
2. Stop smoking
3. Be more physically active
4. Eat a healthier diet

Your risk of developing most types of cancer can be significantly reduced by changes in your lifestyle. Number one: if you smoke or use tobacco, quit. Number two: when you're in the sun, protect your skin (limited exposure is good because you need vitamin D). Number three: get physically active. And number four: eat better, because a healthy diet reduces your chances of cancer. Those are simple, common sense things that you can do on your own behalf. We'll be covering these items in greater detail as we go.

Just as critical is your yearly physical, and recommended cancer screenings and tests. Don't put off these tests because you're too busy or it's uncomfortable or embarrassing. Often times, we can catch cancer or pre-cancerous conditions early before they become health-threatening.

Take a look at the list of the nine most common forms of cancer. See a trend? They are cancers that can often be avoided or treated if you take the right precautions and commit to getting your exams for early detection. With cancer, ignorance is not bliss—it's deadly. Please decide today to do everything you can to be cancer-free.

✚ OTHER COMMON CHRONIC ILLNESSES

Other chronic illnesses that top the danger list are high blood pressure, respiratory diseases like asthma and emphysema, and Alzheimer's. These are the health conditions that we really have to work hard on preventing and minimizing.

Here's a startling statistic: according to the Alzheimer's Association, every 70 seconds another person develops

Alzheimer's. By mid-century, someone will develop the disease every 33 seconds.[11]

All right, all right—enough doom and gloom. The silver lining is that many of these illnesses are preventable. Yes, really! There is much we can do to take our health into our own hands. In fact, every time you pick up this book, I want you to congratulate yourself because the doctor in the mirror is taking your health into your own hands. The upcoming pages are filled with ideas, tips, and strategies that can improve the quality and longevity of your life—they should end up dog-eared and filled with Post-it® Notes as you read and reread them over the years. Just like your body shouldn't spend too much time sitting around collecting dust, neither should this book.

✚ BONUS YEARS

How does a person promote health and prevent disease and live beyond the average life expectancy? After all, do you consider yourself average? The majority of Americans think they are above average, which doesn't make mathematical sense, but it fits perfectly with our indomitable spirit. And to tell the truth, the qualities of high spirit and optimism are proven to extend lives.

Let's say you want to live longer than the national average of 78.[12] This is called reaching the "bonus years," and it is

DR. YOU MEDICAL NOTE:

Want to increase your chances of living longer? Be a "glass half full" person. Reports say you could add 7.5 bonus years to your life.

an important goal. But, as you know, you have to give a little to get a little. What are you willing to do to get your bonus years? Maybe it's a relatively small change to your diet. Eat more raw vegetables at lunch, for example. That won't kill you. It may, in fact, do the exact opposite.

Or you could take up a sport like golf or tennis. That's like getting double points because you'll be gaining both exercise and camaraderie, two factors that help older adults reach the bonus years.

Or how about volunteer work? That will increase your activity level and your amount of socialization—again, two key contributors to a longer life. I like to say that volunteering can be a lifesaver for you, as well as for the people you're serving.

There is one secret of centenarians (those who live beyond 100) that all of us can incorporate into our lives. It doesn't cost a cent. You don't need a lick of athletic ability or any special "tofu genes." And you can use this secret anytime, any place. What is it? Be a "glass half full" person. No kidding. One of the secrets to living longer is a positive outlook. You might think that's a bunch of hogwash, but studies have shown it to be true.

Being a "glass half full" person can make you more resilient to illness. It can lower your blood pressure. It typically makes you more proactive about health issues, too. I've seen studies that report being positive adds 7.5 years to life.[13] All of that in a simple positive outlook. That's some pretty powerful medicine in that half-glass. Cheers!

✚ HEALTHY IS PATRIOTIC

These days, you can't flip on the television or radio or read a newspaper without someone telling you (usually in a loud voice) who is or who is not patriotic. Such commentary is especially commonplace in the political arena, and politics is a place I'll steer clear of. Except to say this: everyone has a right to their opinions. Let's just agree to be informed and respectful in our discussions. (And best not at the dinner table.) And, if it's appropriate to your views and your community's circumstances, you should consider supporting public policies that bolster health initiatives.

What I will say about patriotism is something you probably have not heard before: *being healthy is patriotic.* Yep. Here's why: Medicare is the third-largest program in our government's budget, after defense spending and social security.[14] Experts agree that with the way the costs are growing, Medicare will soon be the largest line item in our budget. That means in the near future, the federal government will be spending more on protecting your health than on protecting the safety of our country.

"Americans need to understand there is a connection between the skyrocketing cost of health care and our lifestyle choices."

You might say, "Sure, but it's not really me that's the problem." We Americans need to understand there is a connection between the skyrocketing cost of health care and our lifestyle choices. I implore you: control what you can control. You need to make healthier lifestyle choices, starting today. Not only for your own sake, but for the sake of your country. Think of it as doing your part.

Here's a flashback to grade school social studies. Medicare was signed into law in July of 1965. Do you know who received the first Medicare card? Harry S. Truman, a darn patriotic guy. But here's the rub. In 1965, the average American life expectancy was about 67 years. That meant, on average, those who were 65 when Medicare began, would receive about two years of federal health insurance coverage before passing away. Two years!

Today, not only is the number of Americans 65-plus booming, but the double whammy is that life expectancies have

DR. YOU MEDICAL NOTE:

Harry S. Truman, received the very first Medicare card. The buck stopped with him. Now the buck needs to stop with you.

increased, too. The average American today lives to be about 78 years old (even though we can do better). So rather than two years of Medicare coverage, now, on average, Americans receive approximately 13 years of coverage. It has become obvious, as life expectancies and our older population continue to rise, and the number of chronic illnesses per person increase, too, that the strain on the system needs to be lightened. This can happen, one healthy Dr. You at a time.

Here's a hard look at some numbers that will help you understand why healthy is patriotic. Currently, the United States spends more money on the health of a 65-year-old than any other country in the world. How do we show our appreciation? As discussed earlier, we've slipped to where 49 countries now have life expectancies that exceed ours. More money, less healthy. That doesn't add up.

What kind of financial hole are our bad health habits digging us into? In 2008, almost one-third ($368.1 billion) of total health care expenditures were spent on care and treatment of the elderly. That's more than seven times as much as we spend on public elementary and secondary education.[15] Cigarette

> **DR. YOU MEDICAL NOTE:**
>
> In 2008, almost one-third ($368.1 billion) of total health care expenditures were spent on care and treatment of the elderly. That's more than seven times as much as we spend on public elementary and secondary education.

smoking costs $96 billion in health care expenditures, with $10 billion more for death- and illness-related expenditures associated with secondhand smoke.[16]

"The United States spends more money on the health of a 65-year-old than any other country in the world"

If you're worried about your grandchildren because the national debt is expanding out of control, think of our expanding national waistline. Obesity-related health costs are growing faster than any previous health issue the nation has faced. If current trends continue, 43% of our population will be considered obese by 2018, costing approximately $344 billion a year.[17] How is that fair?

If you want to do something for your country, for yourself, and for your grandchildren, turn off the TV and walk around the block a few times each day. Cut that bowl of ice cream in half. Get out and be active in the community rather than grumbling from the easy chair. Those are things you can control. That's being healthy. That's being patriotic.

DOCTOR'S ORDERS
HEALTH IN AMERICA

- Recognize that Dr. You is one of your very best health advocates.

- America is lagging behind many nations in critical health indicators, including being a dismal 50th in life expectancy.

- Don't fool yourself that poor health is "normal aging."

- Watch out for the big three chronic diseases: arthritis, cardiovascular disease, and cancer.

- Increase your chances of living 7.5 years longer with a glass-half-full attitude.

- Do your part. Being healthy is being patriotic as over 200,000 Americans age into Medicare each month—putting an unprecedented strain on the program.

- We all pay the price of each other's unhealthy lifestyle decisions.

Dr. You

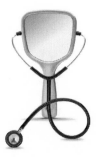

CHAPTER 2

BAD HABITS

✚ ARE YOUR CHOICES KILLING YOU?

Right now is as good a time as any to set some ground rules for this book. Take a look in the mirror and begin by envisioning the healthiest possible you. What does he or she look like? What can this vision of you do? Where does your healthiest possible you go and whom do you see?

The million-dollar question is how do you take control of your health and become this person? The answer: one penny at a time. Beginning with deciding to love, appreciate, and

DR. YOU MEDICAL NOTE:

Most chronic illnesses affecting those 60-plus are a direct result of behavior.

value yourself, to care more about yourself, and to make better choices. It's time to become more deeply invested in your health.

Don't get me wrong; some medical conditions are unpreventable and beyond your control. For any such illness, you have to focus on what you can control: your reaction to it. That is, how you can make yourself stronger "around the illness."

Earlier we mentioned that there are several types of arthritis. Say, for example, you have rheumatoid arthritis. This is an inflammation of the joints and surrounding tissues that can also affect organs and all aspects of life. Oftentimes, it is hereditary. So where's the control in that? I've had the pleasure of knowing some pretty special people who have taught me that the control is in how you make yourself stronger around the illness. Physical therapy, strengthening exercises, and medication can delay and lessen the debilitating effects of rheumatoid arthritis. Your response plays a critical role in your future. If you decide, "I was dealt a lousy hand of cards; I'm going to fold," your life will reflect that negative response. But if you decide to draw a few new cards and play on, good things can happen.

Your behavior will positively or negatively affect your condition.

LEADING FACTORS OF PREMATURE DEATH IN SENIORS

1. 50% Behavior
2. 20% Environment
3. 20% Genetics
4. 10% Access

The point is that even though heredity or fate sometimes deals us a hand we have trouble overcoming, we almost always have some choice in how debilitating the condition becomes, or the effect it has on our overall quality of life.

The good news is that to an extraordinary degree, YOU have control over your health status. As a rule, most of the deadly diseases afflicting those 60-plus are a direct result of behavior. Did you get that? Here's where, as a doctor, I am obligated to repeat myself to make sure this important finding is clear: most of the deadly diseases afflicting those 60-plus are a direct result of behavior.

That means most of the time you have no one to blame but yourself. Pretty harsh statement, you might think. I don't mean to be negative, but I learned long ago that good doctors don't try to win popularity contests. I have to win your attention, your respect, and your trust. That's how this book is going to become a life-changer for you. If I'm completely honest with you, then Dr. You can be completely honest with you, too. That's how barriers are broken down and you become healthier.

But I also believe in the power of positive treatment. My honesty with you will always come in a positive manner. Those are the ground rules.

Let's look at some eye-opening statistics: of the leading causes of death, 50% of the time, *personal behavior* is the key contributor.[1] What makes up the other half of the picture? Let's say you have poor *access* to a regular source of health care because of financial constraints or where you live; ten percent of the time, *access* is a key contributor to cause of death. *Genetics*: 20% of the time. And if you live in an unhealthy or dangerous city or community, or have a dangerous or unhealthy job, 20% of the time those *environmental factors* are key contributors to the leading causes of death.

But don't forget, when it comes to the factors out of your direct control, say, for example, an unhealthy work environment, don't remain an innocent victim. There are ways for you to reach out and talk with your employer about safety issues concerning you. One starting place for more information is the Occupational Safety & Health Administration (OSHA). Find them at www.osha.gov.

But far and away, personal behavior, at around 50%, is the key contributor to the leading causes of death. I call this "causes and consequences." Meaning, if you do this, chances are greatly increased that as a consequence, you will develop a chronic illness that will lead to death.

Take, for example, the leading cause of death for seniors: cardiovascular disease (CVD). What behaviors or risk factors substantially increase your chances of being stricken by CVD? Tobacco use, poor diet, physical inactivity, diabetes, high blood pressure, and high cholesterol. Unfortunately, all these risk factors remain at persistently high levels, or are getting worse. How many of these risk factors apply to you? Every one of those factors can be moderated or eliminated in the creation of the healthiest you. The choice is yours!

Let's look at the most lethal risk factors one at a time. These are the biggies. The behaviors that pile up on you, more than endangering your health—they turn you into a walking time bomb.

+ THE SMOKING GUN

Smoking accounts for an estimated 443,000 deaths each year in the U.S. That's nearly one in every five deaths.[2, 3] Almost one in five — wow. We've all heard numbers like this before, but to what effect? Big, impersonal numbers can be hard to visualize and apply to everyday life, making them ineffective educators.

DEADLY CHOICES

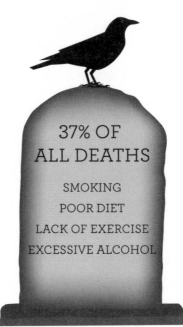

37% OF
ALL DEATHS

SMOKING
POOR DIET
LACK OF EXERCISE
EXCESSIVE ALCOHOL

Here's how I'd like you to remember how lethal cigarette smoking is, especially those of you who smoke. Let's say you smoke with your right hand. Hold that hand out (lefties use your left). Chances are you have five fingers on that hand. Now, fold your index finger down. That's a graphic representation of what one in five deaths looks like. The next time you go to smoke, keep that index finger folded down; that finger is gone, it's dead, so you can't use it. Try pulling, lighting, and holding a cigarette without your index finger. Really, I dare you. Try enjoying a cigarette with only four fingers. Chances are you can't, and that's good. You shouldn't be holding a cigarette in the first place!

> **"If you take a permanent vacation from smoking, you'll have permanent money for vacations. How great is that!"**

Despite all the warnings, there has only been a slight decrease in the number of smokers in the past 25 years. An estimated 18.6% of adult Americans still smoke.[4] That's just under one in five (that ratio doesn't want to go away).

Here's the good news. It's never too late to quit smoking. It's plain wrong to think the damage is already done if you've been smoking for 30 or 40 years. Benefits can begin in as little as 20 minutes! Immediate health improvements include better breathing, circulation, and sleep. Expect to encounter less coughing, fewer illnesses, and more energy. Food and drink taste better as your senses rebound after being dulled by smoking. Plus you and your clothes don't reek of nasty cigarette smoke anymore. And you'll no longer be the source of dangerous secondhand smoke. It goes like this: one small positive change leads to another to another, and suddenly the change you experience is large.

Just imagine the money you'll save by quitting smoking. A one-pack-per-day smoker spends around $1800 per year on his or her habit. And that price tag is only going up. Think of it like this: if you take a permanent vacation from smoking, you'll have permanent money for vacations. How great is that!

Need one last motivator? The youth of America. When kids see Grandma and Grandpa smoke, your behavior is telling them it's okay. Youth smoking is an epidemic. Each day in the United States, approximately 3,450 young people between 12 and 17 years of age smoke their first cigarette, and an estimated 850 youth become daily cigarette smokers.[5] Tragically, between one-third and one-half of those will eventually die as a result of their addiction.[6] Also, secondhand smoke kills an estimated 50,000 people a year.[7] Young children are especially vulnerable; secondhand smoke causes higher risk for a variety of illnesses such as asthma, pneumonia, ear infections, and sudden infant death syndrome.

Be a great role model. Don't smoke, and don't pass it or its effects on to the next generation. You'll be creating a healthier you, a healthier family, and a healthier world.

✚ OBESITY HAS BECOME IMPOSSIBLE TO IGNORE

During my travels throughout the country, I spend many hours in airports, waiting for flights, watching America walk by. I must say, sometimes it's a downright depressing sight. Obesity has become as common as a carry-on bag—in fact, it is our carry-on bag.

Obesity occurs when an excessive amount of body fat accumulates, making a person's weight much greater than normal.

DR. YOU MEDICAL NOTE:

Obesity has more than doubled for people ages 55 to 74. An adult who has a BMI of 30 or above is considered obese.

Typically, obesity is caused by consistently consuming more calories than are burned off.

Obesity can be determined by calculating your body mass index (BMI), a measure of your body fat, based on height and weight. The National Heart, Lung and Blood Institute has a simple-to-use calculator on their website. Go to www.nhlbisup-port.com/bmi/ and find out where you rate (underweight; normal; overweight; obese).

For the more technically savvy, you can download an app on your smartphone to help you and others calculate their BMI. Just be tactful in your approach on this subject: "Excuse me, can I calculate your body mass index to see if you're obese?" is not a particularly good conversation starter.

If you want to test not only your body mass index but also your math skills, here's how to calculate BMI with a pencil and paper. Take your weight in pounds multiplied by 703 and divide that by your height in inches squared. If your number comes back under 18.5 you're underweight. Normal weight is 18.5 to 24.9. Overweight is 25 to 29.9. Obesity is a BMI of 30 or above.

DR. YOU MEDICAL NOTE:

To calculate your body mass index (BMI) go to
www.nhlbisupport.com/bmi.
Obesity is a BMI of 30 or above.

Here's a heart-breaking statistic. According to the Centers for Disease Control, approximately 39% of people ages 55 to 74 are obese. Since 1980, obesity among this age group has more than doubled. We are now on track for obesity to overtake smoking as the number one cause of preventable death. How do we, as our country's senior citizens, account for this? How can we just go on happily eating ourselves into an early grave?

A new report from University of Minnesota researchers suggests that the vast majority of obese Americans do not think their weight problems translate into poor health.[8] This type of denial is frightening. It has to end here and now. The health risks of obesity are unquestionable. To name a few: heart disease, stroke, diabetes, arthritis, cancer, and high blood pressure are linked to this epidemic. Take, for example, obesity-related cancers. Obesity can cause elevated insulin levels, and excess insulin is believed to fuel the growth of cancer cells. More and more studies are also showing a link between obesity and a weakened immune system, and even a link to Alzheimer's disease.

"Healthy progress can become more addictive than the unhealthy food that caused the problem in the first place."

We'll discuss in the upcoming pages numerous simple, practical tips and strategies around diet and exercise that can help fight obesity. There are also surgical procedures such as bariatric surgery (reducing the size of the stomach), but that procedure is generally not recommended past age 65.

Here's one of the underlying problems of obesity: nearly one in three American adults are obese—more than 66 million men and women—so it's easy to get fooled that this is the new normal. You may find yourself saying, "Hey, I don't look that different from my sister, so my weight is not such a big deal." What researchers have found is that obesity can spread in social circles, and the closer the connection you have with a person who is obese, the greater the influence can be on developing obesity. Look at these research findings:[9]

- A person's chances of becoming obese increased by 57% if he or she had a close friend who became obese.

- In same-sex friendships, a close friend becoming obese increased the chances of becoming obese by 71%. However, no such association was found in opposite-sex friendships.

- The perception of friendship also was an important factor. When two people identified each other as close friends, the risk of one person becoming obese increased by 171% if his or her friend became obese.

- Among pairs of siblings, one becoming obese increased the other's chance of becoming obese by 40%. This finding was more marked among same-sex siblings than opposite-sex siblings.

- In married couples, one spouse becoming obese increased the likelihood of the other spouse becoming obese by 37%. Husbands and wives appeared to affect each other equally.

The bottom line is that obesity is making our nation's population sicker than at any time the history of our country. Furthermore, our social circles have a great effect on our overall health. In a way, unhealthy behavior by a close friend or family member can give you "false permission" for your own unhealthy behavior. Don't fall prey to that influence.

It's time for Dr. You to look in the mirror, and as a good doctor will do, be honest about what's happening. We don't want to be remembered as the obese generation, right? Let's start anew, beginning today.

First, using scientific measures, calculate your body mass index to determine what weight category you're in. Then, make a plan for getting your weight down to a healthier level (or maintaining a healthy level). Not in a few months through fad diets or miracle weight-loss supplements, but over a healthy, safe, extended period of time. Maybe a pound of fat every month or two.

The good news is that your progress can become more addictive than the unhealthy food that caused the problem in the first place. And if it is indeed true that weight goes on easier if you're surrounded by unhealthy behavior, then it stands to

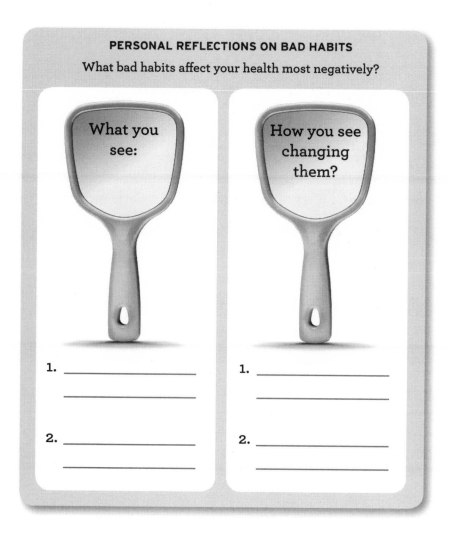

PERSONAL REFLECTIONS ON BAD HABITS
What bad habits affect your health most negatively?

What you see:

How you see changing them?

1. _____
   _____

2. _____
   _____

1. _____
   _____

2. _____
   _____

reason it comes off easier if you're surrounded by healthy groups of friends. Partner up with a loved one or friend and begin taking off unhealthy weight together.

In chapter four, we will talk more about the power of exercising in a group. You'll hear the story of how entire communities in Louisville, Seattle, and Oklahoma City are on their way to shedding millions of pounds in citywide programs. (For a sneak peek see www.thiscityisgoingonadiet.com.) You can start losing unhealthy weight, too. Others in similar situations have, and have reported they have a new lease on life.

✚ BE CAREFUL OF ALCOHOL

Maybe you're thinking, "C'mon Dr. Reed. Don't be such a fuddy-duddy. I want to live a little." Well, believe me, I want you to do more than live a little. I want you to live a lot. And the best way to make that happen is to keep this book (and your mind) open, and really read the pages, and really let the message sink in. Then and only then can you make a plan that gets you thinking and living healthier.

Does that mean you can never have a cold beer, a glass of wine, or a cocktail along with a lean cut of steak? No, it does not. You've worked hard for two-thirds of your life, so you deserve to enjoy the life ahead. As I like to tell people, "This is your time!" But enjoyment and an unhealthy lifestyle are not to be confused as the same thing. An occasional serving of lean meat? That's not an unhealthy lifestyle. A glass of wine with dinner? That can be heart healthy. Moderation. Balance. Those are the messages that that the doctor in the mirror needs to keep encouraging.

"A glass of wine with dinner? That can be heart healthy. Moderation and balance are the messages that the doctor in the mirror needs to keep encouraging."

You already know that alcohol in excess is unhealthy and dangerous. Additionally, it is a central-nervous system depressant that can slow your metabolism, causing your body to burn calories less efficiently (remember that when trying to lose weight). Speaking of calories, alcohol is loaded with what we call "empty calories," meaning it has poor nutritional value and provides your body with little or no energy. It also affects judgment, coordination, and inhibition. Heavy alcohol use will raise your blood pressure, and it's linked to obesity, prostate cancer, liver disease, breast cancer, and other diseases. It is also frequently paired with other unhealthy behaviors like smoking and poor eating habits.

As you age, you can become more sensitive to the effects of alcohol. Suddenly you could be slurring words or getting tipsy (literally), when previously the same amount of alcohol had a lesser effect.

Always be careful about mixing alcohol with prescription meds. It can interfere with the effectiveness of your medication, and worse, lead to unwanted side effects or dangerous reactions. Even though the label may carry a clear warning, we see people going to emergency rooms every day because they mixed alcohol and medication. Please, don't be one of those people.

My bottom line: before bottoms up, keep in mind that the danger of alcohol is not to be underestimated—it is to be respected. Alcohol in moderation is fine. There is no scientific definition for moderate drinking, but it is generally defined as no more than one drink per day for women, and no more than two drinks per day for men. This definition is intended for single-day consumption, by the way, and not to be averaged out over several days.

All of us want to live a little. I say, let's shoot higher. When we do things right, we can live a lot.

+ THE SEDENTARY LIFE

Back when many of us were young adults and just getting on our feet with jobs and family, our society had cultivated a romantic, idyllic view of what to expect in the latter part of life:

DR. YOU MEDICAL NOTE:

Currently, 44% of people 65-plus are considered "inactive," meaning they engage in less than 10 minutes of moderate or vigorous activity weekly.

sitting around, doing nothing but full-time relaxing. That would be the good life, right? Let me tell you, if you sit around all day and do nothing, there is nothing idyllic nor romantic about what happens to you.

> "Some doctors and researchers have gone so far as to call sitting the new smoking."

One of the most unhealthy practices we've gotten into as a country in the last half-century is to sink into a sedentary lifestyle. The word sedentary comes from the Latin *sedentrius* or sedere, meaning "to sit." Want to know my translation for sedentary? Couch potato. Again, not a very idyllic image. Far too many older Americans are getting little to no regular physical activity. Currently, 44% of adults 65-plus are considered "inactive," meaning they engage in less than ten minutes of moderate or vigorous activity weekly. Ten minutes. Weekly! Literally, the word sedentary couldn't be more appropriate; we sit way too much. Some doctors and researchers have gone so far as to call sitting the new smoking.

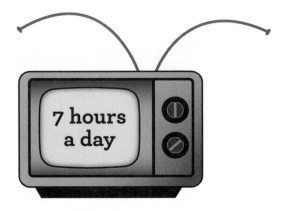

Older adults watch too much TV

Our current culture is wired for sedentary behavior—or should I say wireless for sedentary behavior, what with all the high-tech gadgets we have. For someone 65-plus, the average time spent daily sitting in front of the TV is about seven hours. [10] The average time spent per day sitting on the Internet is almost two hours.[11] What's more, TV and computers are magnets for unhealthy snacks. How many times have you brought "just one more bowl" into the TV room or to your computer desk? Add to that the comfort of air-conditioned cars to take us a few blocks here and there, and it's no wonder our legs are so inactive—remember, your largest muscles are in your legs, so if you want to get your metabolism burning calories, those are the muscles to get in gear.

So, in the spirit of better health through better habits, I'm going to ask you to get up and read the rest of this chapter while standing. Just a couple of minutes or so. (No, this time I'm not kidding.) If you like to read, occasionally get up and do so while standing. Or during the commercial break of your television program, do some toe touches and deep-knee bends.

Just think about how many times over the course of your life you're going to need to get up and out of a chair; by turning moments of downtime into uptime now, inactivity will take less of a toll on you later. Studies show just a minute on your feet gets your body and metabolism going. Seriously, all the sitting is unhealthy.

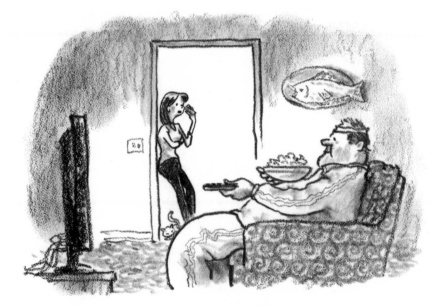

"John's doing a marathon today.
Unfortunately it's one of those 24-hour Western marathons."

> **"Remember, you're a part of the human race, not the human sit."**

A University of South Carolina study of middle-aged men found that those who sat more than 23 hours a week—watching TV or sitting in a car—had a far greater risk of cardiovascular disease than those who sat less than 11 hours.[12]

Remember, you're part of the human race, not the human sit. Let's get up and get active. Every little bit counts.

Are you still standing?

✚ HIGH BLOOD PRESSURE: THE SILENT KILLER

High blood pressure isn't what you'd call a bad habit, but often, it's the result of them. Several factors are thought to cause high blood pressure, including smoking, being overweight, lack of physical activity, and overconsumption of sodium and alcohol.

Also known as hypertension, high blood pressure doesn't refer to being stressed or tense; in fact, you can be cool as a cucumber and still have dangerously high blood pressure. What few people realize (until it's too late) is that high blood pressure usually has no outward symptoms. That is why it's known as the "silent killer."

As you probably know, there are two numbers used in a blood pressure reading. For example, the generally accepted optimal blood pressure for an adult is 120/80 mmHg (mmHg is millimeters of mercury). Typically, 120/80 is read "one-twenty over eighty," but as the doctor in the mirror, do you know what those numbers mean? This is important stuff that you need to know in order to be hale and hearty.

The top number is the *systolic* reading, and it's a measurement of the force exerted by the heart against the blood vessels when it pumps blood to the body. The bottom number is the *diastolic* reading, and it's a measurement of the pressure when the heart is at rest between beats.

Over half of all Americans age 60-plus have high blood pressure, which means they have a reading of 140/90 or higher. But statistics estimate that only 44% are treated to get their blood pressure to the right levels. High blood pressure can lead to stroke, heart attack, heart failure, kidney disease, and eye damage, as well as increasing the likelihood of cardiovascular disease related sickness and death. This is serious stuff, folks.

Of course both the higher *systolic* number and lower *diastolic* number are very important. But newer guidelines are telling doctors to pay the greatest attention to the systolic pressure—especially for adults 50 and over.

How in the world are you going to remember all of this blood pressure information? As an eminent geriatrician once told me, "You can't learn what you can't remember." Try this memory trick:

Healthy BP s̲hould add up to 200.

The s in s̲hould comes first, and is underlined, because it stands for systolic blood pressure: the reading that comes first when your blood pressure is tested. The d in shoul̲d comes last, and is underlined, because it stands for diastolic blood pressure: the reading that comes last when your blood pressure is tested.

Healthy BP s̲houl̲d add up to 200.

Read it over a few times and you'll have it for life. Speaking of life, don't forget to have your blood pressure checked this year. Did you know that most fire stations do it for free? What better reason to stop in and tell these men and women what an admirable service they provide.

✚ NEED ATTITUDE REPLACEMENT SURGERY?

One of the most serious conditions affecting the health of folks 55-plus is something that can be completely controlled by those suffering from it. It's called, in highly technical medical terms, a cruddy attitude. I talked earlier in the book about "glass half full" people and how a positive mindset has been calculated to add 7.5 years to a life. Well folks, it's time you got healthier by ridding yourself of one of the worst habits since deep-fried cheese curds: negativity.

"The worst health habit since deep-fried cheese curds is a negative attitude."

I think the doctor in the mirror could prescribe a little attitude adjustment. Or if your attitude has been really negative lately, you might be a candidate for attitude replacement surgery.

Did you know that there's this thing on the front of your face, maybe you've heard of it? It's crescent-shaped … it's called a smile. Have you seen yours lately? It's a sign of good health.

Now, I know what some of you are thinking: "Dr. Reed, you don't know diddly-squat about what I've been through. You don't know how I hurt. You don't know the situation I'm in." I respect that; you're right. Dr. You knows you better than anyone. But we all face tremendous challenges, illness, and hardship in this life—some more than others Every person has a decision to make: am I going to be a victim or a survivor? A positive attitude can be the difference-maker.

Dear Reader, I want to share something I've learned with you. I've spent over 40 years passionately listening, observing, and caring for the health needs of good people just like you. Currently, thanks to my position with UnitedHealth Group, I have what I refer to as 70 million patients. As the Chief of Medical Affairs, I get to work with thousands of talented professionals dedicated to finding effective, exciting ways to help the people we serve live healthier lives. It's a privilege to consult with so many amazing health care professionals, as well as work with such a wealth of information — especially regarding older adults. My point is, one key fact keeps popping up over and over and over again: turning a negative attitude into a positive attitude has tremendous health benefits.

Maybe you or a loved one is stubborn. Believe me, I've dealt with that. I constantly hear people say things like, "Somebody my age can't do that. I'm too old and set in my ways." That's baloney! You can make amazing progress as long as you don't try to accomplish everything in one day or one week or one month; that's not how human beings work.

Change doesn't happen overnight, it happens over time. This book is about starting with small changes. And no, change isn't easy. You need to allow yourself time to think about it, to begin to see that there is a better way, to set goals. The decision is yours. Understand that it's okay when, occasionally, you take a step backward. Just get it into your head that this change is for the better and you're going to get there. In due time.

Start right now. Make a simple plan for improvement. Pick five health goals and write them down on the chart provided. I even included a chart for myself so you wouldn't feel all alone. Don't overdo it. Don't try to do too much too fast. Slow and steady wins the race.

"Look good, feel good. Guys, get to the barbershop. Ladies, try a new hairstyle."

Here's an example. Maybe your plan includes changing one bad habit. Let's say you love ice cream before bed. Instead of a bowl, put your treat in a coffee cup. That will reduce the serving size. As time goes on, maybe on every other trip to the grocery store, buy frozen yogurt or sherbet as a lower-fat alternative to your cup of ice cream. Suddenly, you go to bed feeling pretty darn good about yourself; you've accomplished something.

Remember, accomplishment is addictive. You know the feeling.

Or let's say your plan to create a more positive attitude includes being a little prouder of your appearance. Guys, get to the barbershop regularly. I know it costs a couple bucks, but hey, the barber has to make a living, and you'll look and feel sharper. Plus you'll get out and about, socializing—that stuff makes a difference in your health.

FIVE HEALTH GOALS

My health goals

1.

2.

3.

4.

5.

DR. REED'S HEALTH GOALS

1. Ride my bike for long distances at competitive speeds

2. Be fit enough to hike to inspirational locations to take photographs

3. Eat a healthy diet to maintain a low BMI so I feel good, and so my clothes fit well

4. Get more sleep so I'm fully engaged when awake

5. Be around to see my grandkids grow into the extraordinary people they are destined to be

---

Ladies, you too. Go have your hair done, and your nails too, while you're at it. Who cares if your husband doesn't notice, others will. The doctor in the mirror will. You're doing things that will make you a little prouder of your appearance, and yourself. That's not vain, that's gussying up your positive attitude.

Coming up, we're going to go over how your diet and activity levels can be improved in your quest to make the years in front of you the best they can be. Some of those bad habits, we're going to break. Some of them we'll only bend. But it's progress. It's a little at a time. Like I love to say, the way to feeling like a million bucks is a penny at a time.

DOCTOR'S ORDERS
BAD HABITS

R$_X$

- Don't allow bad habits to get in the way of becoming the person you always hoped to be.

- Most deadly diseases afflicting those 60-plus are a direct result of behavior.

- Beware of smoking, poor diet, a sedentary lifestyle, and alcohol abuse, as they are leading risk factors of deadly diseases.

- Quit smoking cigarettes. Smoking accounts for nearly one in five deaths.

- Watch your weight. 39% of the people ages 55 to 74 are obese. Since 1980, obesity among this age group has more than doubled.

- Don't sit your life away. Forty-four percent of adults 65-plus are considered "inactive," because they engage in less than ten minutes of moderate or vigorous activity weekly.

- Have your blood pressure checked regularly; high blood pressure can have no outward symptoms, which is why it's called the "silent killer."

- Little improvements add up in a big way. The way to feeling like a million bucks is a penny at a time.

Dr. You

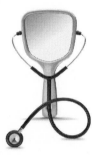

CHAPTER 3

HEALTHY DIET

✚ KNOWLEDGE IS POWERFUL FOOD

Folks, to become an outstanding doctor in the mirror, you need to learn about something that we often do without thinking at all: eat. I don't know if you can identify with this, but sometimes when we open our mouths to eat, it seems to shut off our brains. For example, what did you have for dinner last night? Or, for that matter, for breakfast this morning?

In this chapter, we're going to think about our food. We will become more knowledgeable about what we eat and drink.

DR. YOU MEDICAL NOTE:

Think of "diet" as a long-term lifestyle change, not a short-term fad.

Don't worry, I'm not talking about you becoming a nutrition-ist and running a lab in your kitchen. I'm much more practical than that. What I'm talking about is getting the basics down. Stuff about food and nutrition that, quite frankly, few of our parents learned, so they never taught it to us. And then with the basics in hand, you can apply that information to change your behavior.

> **"When we open our mouths to eat, it seems to shut off our brains."**

I am asking you to come into this chapter with a willing-ness to change. I know that's easier said than done. (I have a few ratty old t-shirts that my wife would love to see tossed out with the trash.) But really, change can be for the better. I talk to people all the time who think change is too restric-tive, that all the flavor will get cut from life. Not true. Change can be fun. And certainly being healthy is a lot more fun than being sick.

DR. YOU MEDICAL NOTE:

Research shows that about 40% of overweight Americans think that they're in the normal range for weight.

So how do you learn what's what about food and diet and nutrition? We live in a time with tremendous access to information. This allows you to get a little smarter about your health and your diet every day. As a reward, you can get a little more out of each day. And that can lead to a life of greater quality and longevity. Pretty soon, you're a very wise person indeed.

Hippocrates, the Greek physician often considered the father of Western medicine, said, "Let food be your medicine and your medicine be your food." Well there's another pretty wise person for you. He figured out long ago that health and food are inseparable.

I'd like you to make a change—right now. Don't let yourself go through life not thinking—or being ignorant—about food. Food and drink are the fuel that runs the miraculous machine known as you. Learn. Try new things. Be open. Knowledge is powerful food.

✚ LET'S TALK ABOUT DIET, THE NOUN

When I use the word diet, I'm almost always using it as a noun. As in: your *diet* is the food and drink that you regularly consume.

Another way to use the word is as a verb. As in: I've been *dieting* for months to lose weight. I'm not a fan of the word diet as a verb. Because study after study shows that when a person is dieting, his or her weight tends to yo-yo down and up. Typically, the only permanent result is frustration.

> **"A calorie is not a measurement of weight. A calorie is a unit of energy."**

Said another way, diet—the noun—is a long-term lifestyle decision. Diet, the verb, is a short-term reactionary decision. Let's figure out how you can create a nutritious, healthy, long-term diet that keeps you going strong for years and years. It's a lifestyle thing. Not a fad thing.

✚ YOU ARE WHAT YOU EAT

If you want to be healthy, consume healthy food and beverages in appropriate amounts. Okay, close the book—we're done.

Well, not so fast. We all know there are numerous barriers out there to eating right. It's time to return to the mirror and identify those barriers. Barriers such as the relatively inexpensive fast food available at nearly every busy intersection and throughout every mall.

DR. YOU MEDICAL NOTE:

The Food and Drug Administration says 2000 calories a day is a reasonable average consumption guideline for most adults.

Sometimes it's difficult to make healthy choices, especially if you're like many Americans today with skimpier paychecks or no paycheck. Maybe you're just getting by on a fixed income, and your monthly social security check can't stretch all the way to the healthy food aisle. Other people tell me that it's hard to find the time to eat right. Gosh, even nutritional guidelines seem to be ever-changing, further complicating things.

Well, complex as it may be, we are going to learn the simple facts, and then put facts into action. Nobody likes a doctor who makes things complicated. So if we're going to be effective, let's boil it down to three simple steps.

First: it's a well-researched fact that diet affects our health and our well-being. It's important that we make the right decisions because, as we've discussed, being overweight or obese increases the likelihood of many chronic and fatal illnesses, including cardiovascular disease, hypertension and stroke, diabetes, osteoarthritis, and several types of cancer.

Second: you need to understand that the old saying "you are what you eat" is true. What fills our plates and cups has so much to do with who we are. When you think of you, do you think of a shiny apple walking down the street? Or maybe a sprig of broccoli dancing? Or a lean piece of fish doing a household chore? Or, on the other hand, do you see a piece of fried chicken slowly making its way down the steps? Or an onion ring snoring on the couch?

Third: if you're going to change, it's important to understand that *how* you think of yourself plays a critical role. Research shows that about 40% of overweight Americans think that they're in the normal range for weight. That's an awful lot of people fooling themselves, which is dangerous because if you don't think there's a problem, why would you think to fix it? We need to take a harder look in the mirror, not only to become the doctor in the mirror, but also to recognize the doctor in the meal, too.

"Are you more like a shiny apple walking down the street, or an onion ring snoring on the couch?"

Let's get going in a positive direction. Let's figure out a way to your healthy, delicious diet, in the right portions, eaten at the right times, in balanced courses. In the end, you will discover that yes, you can have your cake and eat it too. Let's just make it a small slice of carrot cake, for starters.

✚ FOOD ENERGY

Let's start with the basic facts: your goal is to create a healthy, energy-rich diet that is nutritious and delicious.

The energy in food is measured in calories. Many people think that a calorie is a measurement of weight. It's not. A calorie is a measurement of a unit of energy. So calories are good; we need energy.

As far as weight gain is concerned, a calorie is a calorie is a calorie; just don't consume more calories than you expend. Be on the lookout for calorie-dense foods that contain many calories but provide minimal vitamins and minerals needed to maintain health. For example, there are only <u>four</u> calories in a gram of protein or carbohydrates. There are <u>seven</u> calories in a gram of alcohol. There are <u>nine</u> calories in a gram of fat. Lesson: one gram can have vastly different calorie implications.

A simple start to a healthy diet is to eat foods that are less calorie-dense. Try this switch-a-roo: instead of a bowl of ice cream, have a few spoonfuls. Instead of a few spoonfuls of fruits and vegetables, have a bowl full.

✚ GUIDELINES FOR YOUR HEALTHY DIET

Now let's translate simple facts into personally appropriate action. To start, you need to know how many daily calories are healthy for you. How much fat? How many carbohydrates?

And by the way, what the heck is a carbohydrate anyhow?

Without getting overly scientific (because few of us have a scientist handy when eating), I will set out some general rules for how Dr. You can start putting together a healthy diet. I want you to have a solid starting point from which to build, based on averages for people age 55-plus.

The risk in doing this is that we're talking about a broad spectrum of people, few of whom actually fit the definition of average. Your specific age, gender, race, height, weight, health condition, and activity level are different from the next person's. But, as I like to say, you have to start somewhere or you'll get nowhere.

Use these guidelines to start a plan for a healthy diet. Be sure to talk to your doctor about your diet. I'll also include online resources to help you individualize your healthy diet.

The Food and Drug Administration says 2000 calories a day is a reasonable average guideline for most adults, so we'll start there. (As you'll soon see, the Nutrition Facts label on food packaging also uses 2000 calories in their daily value calculations. You may need more or less based on your health conditions; consult with your physician or a nutritionist to be sure.) Did you know that the average adult should consume roughly 2000 calories a day? If not, we're already making progress.

As we were growing up—in fact, until very recently—we were encouraged to think about food consumption in terms of

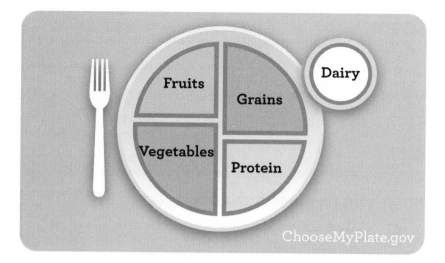

a pyramid. I don't know about you, but I found it to be kind of confusing. Now there's a handy, simpler way, using a plate instead.

Look at the accompanying plate graphic. As a starting point, make half your plate fruits and vegetables. Grains and proteins should make up the other half, with grains being a slightly larger share. Keep your dairy low-fat or fat-free.

Here's a good tip to remember and share with friends and family: you want to eat a "colorful" plate—with fruits and vegetables leading the way. Much of your daily recommended carbohydrates and fiber are in fruits and veggies. Next, make at least half of your grains whole grains. Among other nutrients found in grains, you'll find carbohydrates and important fiber.

Keep your protein lean: fish, skinless poultry, nuts, beans, and lean red meat, to name a few. Remember, low-fat dairy will provide calcium-rich foods important for strong bones and more. And don't forget to count the calories in your beverages.

For more specific food guidance, go to choosemyplate.gov, and type "get a personalized plan" into the search box. You'll get a daily food plan based on your age, sex, weight, and physical activity.

Get a more precise calorie recommendation tailored to you at www.mayoclinic.com/health/calorie-calculator/NU00598.

Web MD has a helpful Food-O-Meter to help you find nutritional information, calories, and portion sizes of many foods and beverages, including those found at fast food restaurants.

> **"Ladies and gentlemen, I'll say it again: knowledge is powerful food."**

✚ THE MIGHTY NUTRITION FACTS

If we're going to make the right healthy eating decisions, we need to know what's in the food we eat and the beverages we drink. To help us with this, dear Reader, I have a surprise for you. Allow me to bring in a guest. Please welcome Margaret Hamburg, MD. In addition to being a Harvard graduate and

> **DR. YOU MEDICAL NOTE:**
>
> Always check for servings per container. Don't assume one package, one serving.

a colleague whose work I know well, she is the Commissioner of the Food and Drug Administration. Very impressive! Here's what Dr. Hamburg said recently: "Today, ready access to reliable information about the calorie and nutrient content of food is even more important, given the prevalence of obesity and diet-related diseases in the United States."

I couldn't have said it better myself. I'm sure you will join me in thanking Dr. Hamburg for her insightful comment, and for her relentless diligence on our behalf for more clarity and openness from the food and beverage companies about what we're eating and drinking.

Because of people like her, gone are the days of, say, mystery meat in a frozen dinner. Thanks to the mighty nutrition label, you now have access to the information you need right on the package to make wise decisions about your diet.

You can compare products on calorie measures, and you can quickly scan important health-related ingredients. That's a big deal because now you can plan how each course fits into the meal, and how each meal fits into a balanced daily 2000-calorie diet. Or, if you're on a specialized or restricted diet, you can literally put your finger on pertinent dietary information so the food and drink you consume fits with your health conditions. Ladies and gentlemen, I'll say it again: knowledge is powerful food.

Why do so many people fail to use this information? Maybe they're just lazy. Maybe the information intimidates them. Maybe they never knew it was there in the first place. Well, we're not going to let that happen to you.

Let's review how to read and use a nutrition label. We'll look at calories per serving, total fat, cholesterol, sodium, and

Use the Nutrition Facts label to eat healthier

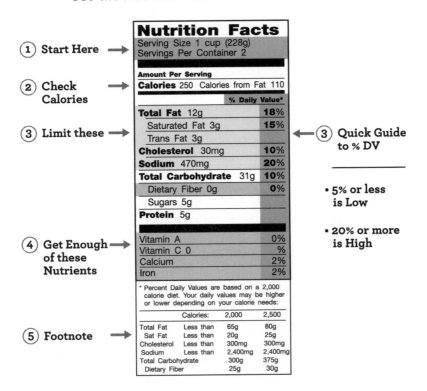

total carbohydrates, including fiber. Know this: being a great label reader is how Dr. You makes sound, healthy diet decisions. Once you get in the habit, you'll find it's fun to find which foods and drinks are the surprise winners and which are the sneaky losers when it comes to nutrition. Seriously. It feels awfully good when you compare—and find—the better choices. Before and after eating them.

✦ UNDERSTANDING "SERVING SIZES"

Much of the information and guidance on a food label is on a per-serving basis. So before you start calculating calories and nutrients (or munching and sipping), make sure that you're aware of the number of servings per container, and the serving size—these are found in the nutrition facts.

Don't assume one package, one serving. That's rarely the case. For example, let's say you have a "friend" who occasionally likes macaroni and cheese. (This is an unhealthy choice, so don't let your "friend" eat it too often.) If the servings per container reads three and the calories per serving is 400 and your friend eats half the box as a side dish with dinner, that "side dish" alone contains 600 calories, or nearly a third of the daily allowance. Frankly, that's the biggest waste of allowance since you broke open your piggy bank and sent away for sea monkeys.

Other times, when the package doesn't list a number of servings, you'll have to visualize a serving size. For example, let's say you plan to put hamburgers on the grill for dinner. Sounds tasty. Your healthy diet calls for one serving of ground beef per patty. What's one serving? You may have grown up in a home where you needed two hands and an elbow to handle "one serving" of your burger. For ground beef, and other red meat, a serving size is about four ounces (or a quarter pound). So, if you have one pound of hamburger, divide it into four parts, and you have four servings. Pretty easy, huh? Well, yes and no. The nutrition and the calories in that hamburger patty can vary based on how lean the meat is, even when the serving size is the same. We will come back to the burger discussion in a few minutes.

APPROXIMATE SINGLE-SERVING SIZES

3 to 4 ounces of meat	Deck of cards
3 to 4 ounces of grilled fish	Checkbook
1 small potato	Computer mouse
1 tablespoon of peanut butter	Tip of your thumb
1 cup of fruit	One baseball
2 cups of mixed greens	Two baseballs
1 cup of raw vegetables	One baseball
¼ cup of dried fruit	Golf ball
1 teaspoon of butter or margarine	One dice (or die)
1 ounce of hard cheese	Two dice
¼ cup of nuts	Palmful

Meanwhile, look at the single-serving chart I have included for you. It has some neat ways to visualize a single serving using household objects. It's not an exact science, but it gets you darn close—and you don't need to be a whiz with a conversion table to do it.

✚ ISN'T FAT BAD?

You wouldn't believe all the people who ask me, "Dr. Reed, how am I supposed to cut all the fat out of my diet?" I always tell them, "I have no idea—because you're not supposed to!"

You see, fat is not the enemy. Fat is essential to life: it is a super-concentrated energy source that helps to fight disease and aids in the absorption of essential vitamins. You might hear or see the words triglycerides or lipids in association with fats. Lipids are a broad group of molecules that include triglycerides. Triglyceride is a medical term for fat.

Most foods contain a combination of different fats. For sure, not all fats are created equal—in fact, they're usually referred to as "bad fats" and "good fats."

Your goal is to get the right amount of "good fats" into your diet and most of the "bad fats" out.

Here's a general rule of thumb to help separate the two in your mind: bad fats are typically solid at room temperature, and they include saturated fat and trans fat. Good fats are typically liquid at room temperature, and they include unsaturated fat such as monounsaturated fat and polyunsaturated fat.

DR. YOU MEDICAL NOTE:

"Bad fats" are typically solid at room temperature, and they include saturated fat and trans fat. "Good fats" are typically liquid at room temperature, and they include unsaturated fat such as monounsaturated fat and polyunsaturated fat.

Now let's return to our good friend the nutrition label. We've covered calories-per-serving. Right below that, you'll see something titled: Total Fat. Take a good look at a few food packages in your pantry and freezer.

The bad fats are saturated fat and trans fat. Most often, saturated fat is found in meat, dairy, fried foods, snack foods, fast food, and rich desserts. Healthy diet guidelines say keep your intake of saturated fat to less than 7% of daily calories.

The most harmful of the bad fats—the evil archenemy of health—is trans fat. (Here's where readers should boo!) Trans fat has a double whammy effect of increasing "bad" cholesterol and decreasing "good" cholesterol. More on that in a second. Most of the trans fats you consume are used to enhance food flavor and keep fat from spoiling quickly. You'll often find trans fat in ingredients such as partially hydrogenated oil, hydrogenated oil, stick margarine, and shortening (as in shortening your life). Limit your intake of trans fat to a little as possible. That means avoiding fried foods, baked goods like cakes and cookies, as well as some crunchy snack foods like chips and crackers containing ingredients from the list above. Check your frozen foods and fast foods, too.

Now let's talk about unsaturated fat or "good fats." There are two types of good fats: polyunsaturated fat and monounsaturated fat. As strange as it may sound, unsaturated fat can actually improve blood cholesterol, which can reduce the risk of heart disease. It can also benefit insulin levels and blood sugar, which can be helpful for diabetes. Good unsaturated fats include olive oil, canola oil, safflower oil, and sunflower oil, to name a few. Omega-3 fatty acid is a type of polyunsaturated fat found in fish like tuna and salmon, plants such as soy, walnuts, seeds, avocados, and to a lesser degree in green vegetables.

As for this final bit of news, I've saved the best for last. Studies show that our very oldest seniors can benefit from a little extra fat. Awesome. That's one more reason to keep on living!

✚ THE RUNAWAY TRAIN CALLED CHOLESTEROL

To function properly, your body needs cholesterol to build cells and certain hormones. Cholesterol is a waxy substance circulating in your blood that comes from two sources: your body and your food. Your liver and other cells make about 75% of the cholesterol in your body. The other 25% comes from the foods you eat.

While cholesterol serves a number of vital roles, high cholesterol in America has become something of a runaway train—a train that leads to obesity and heart disease, among other stops along the way. Consider this: about 43% of men age 55-plus have high cholesterol, as do 51% of women in the same age bracket. [1] Would you have guessed that on average, women have higher cholesterol than men? Regardless of who has it, elevated cholesterol can be a killer.

Rather than continuing to allow dangerously high cholesterol to play a role in the premature death of too many friends and loved ones, vow to do something about it. And that starts with reading the nutrition label. The cholesterol amounts are listed in the next section below the fats. Please, this is vital information that Dr. You needs to know.

In addition to monitoring the amount of cholesterol in your diet, some of you need to be extra vigilant. You may already know you're in the high-risk group, or maybe you're there without your knowledge. Get a simple cholesterol screening during your yearly physical. A small blood sample is drawn and sent to a lab to check for two types of cholesterol, commonly called "good" cholesterol and "bad" cholesterol (just as there were good and bad fats).

Low-density lipoprotein (LDL) is bad cholesterol. Trans fats such as those we just talked about increase LDL, which can slowly build up in the inner walls of your arteries—the major

DR. YOU MEDICAL NOTE:

An estimated 43% of men age 55-plus have high cholesterol, as do 51% of women in the same age bracket.

roadways to the heart and brain. When arteries become too congested, plaque can form, causing thick, hard deposits that narrow the arteries and restrict blood flow to your vital organs. If a clot forms, a heart attack or stroke can result. Most people 55-plus will want to strive for an LDL number of 130 mg/dl (milligrams per deciliter) and below. If you have risk factors for heart disease, your doctor will target a lower number, typically from 70 mg/dl to 100 mg/dl.

The good cholesterol is high-density lipoprotein (HDL). Trans fats rob the body of good cholesterol. One way to remember the difference is look at the first letter of each: HDL is Heavenly and LDL is Lethal.

Studies show that high HDL appears to protect against heart attacks. Experts believe that HDL can remove excess cholesterol and plaque from arteries, in effect cleaning them. A healthy HDL number to strive for is 60 mg/dl and above.

Adding LDL and HDL together, you get your total cholesterol number. Your target number should be 200 mg/dl and below. Common strategies to reduce cholesterol include cutting some unnecessary fats from your diet, especially saturated fat and those good-for-nothing trans fats. Such adjustments, plus exercise, and in some cases medication, can serve to keep your cholesterol levels healthy.

One other number to watch, as we discussed earlier, is your triglycerides: the fat in your diet. Your doctor will usually check your triglycerides during a cholesterol test (sometimes called a lipid profile). Keeping triglycerides low is important to heart health. Coming up shortly, you'll get a worksheet called "Know Your Health in Numbers" for tracking and recording blood pressure, cholesterol, triglycerides and more. The American Heart Association says an optimum triglyceride level is 100 mg/dl.

Friends, read your food labels and be sure to get your cholesterol checked as soon as possible, because often there are no outward signs of dangerously high LDL or dangerously low HDL levels—and we don't want you in danger.

+ PASS THE SODIUM (HAVE LESS, THAT IS)

Next up on the nutrition label is sodium. Everybody knows sodium and salt are the same thing, right? Well, no. Sodium is a type of salt. Table salt, for example, is 40% sodium.

The fact is, in most foods, sodium is naturally present. And not just solid foods. Read beverage labels to monitor how much sodium you're getting in drinks such as soda, malts, and tomato juice; their levels can be high. Which leads me to a tip for

Dr. You: just because it doesn't taste salty doesn't mean it isn't loaded with sodium. Be especially wary of processed foods, as they account for most of the sodium we consume.

"We hardly ever visibly see (and oftentimes don't taste) all the sodium we consume."

It is estimated that nine out of ten Americans get far too much sodium everyday. That is a scary number. Strange thing is, though, only about 5–10% comes from our salt shakers. An estimated 77% comes from the sodium that's loaded into processed foods—like frozen pizza or canned goods—or restaurant meals.[2] If you think about it, that means we hardly ever visibly see all the sodium we're consuming.

You may say, "I never add much salt to food. I don't need to worry about sodium." Well, look out. Because now you know it's already been added (and added and added) for you. What's more, as you age, your taste buds become less sensitive to salt, which can cause folks to add more salt in order to detect a salty taste.

The other day I heard a man who was supposed to be on a strict low-salt diet say that he doesn't use salt, he just fries up some scrapple with his eggs every morning. Of course, if he knew how to read the nutrition facts for sodium like you do

It's estimated that nine out of ten American get far too much sodium every day, but only about 5%–10% comes from our salt shakers.

now, he'd see that his scrapple was loaded with sodium well before it hit the frying pan.

The bottom line is we have to turn on our brains before and when we eat. For example, I had a small whole-wheat bagel for breakfast. Pretty good, right? One gram of fat. Zero cholesterol. Got 24% of my daily dietary fiber. Then, ka-pow! Sodium content: 370 mg! Almost 25% of my daily allotment. In one little whole-wheat bagel that was smaller than my fist. And it didn't taste the least bit salty to me. I'll have to watch my sodium intake for the rest of the day. Also be on the lookout for sauces, condiments such as ketchup, soy sauce, steak sauce, and salad dressing, for example, because they are loaded with sodium.

The lesson is, look at your nutrition labels. Guidelines warn those of us age 51 or over not to exceed 1500 milligrams of sodium per day. Experts say, on average, we're getting twice that much. This is one reason why so many Americans have high blood pressure, putting us at serious risk for heart disease and stroke. How serious is the risk? Analysts estimate that population-wide reductions in sodium could prevent more than 100,000 deaths annually.[3]

What should you do? Again, it gets back to looking at those amazingly helpful nutrition labels. Start to compare and make good choices when you're shopping. And try to really limit trips to the fast food joints. I know, the price is right, and the convenience can't be beat. But you're paying a much larger price than what's listed on the menu board. If you think of the health consequences of eating fast food on a regular basis, the costs in medication, hospitalization, lost time from work or family due to illness—that's the most expensive food on the planet.

One final tip: if you're serving canned vegetables or beans at home, rinse them well with water to remove as much of the sodium as possible.

✚ THE MISUNDERSTOOD CARBOHYDRATE

Our bodies run on things called macronutrients. "Macro" means large, so macronutrients are nutrients that we need in large amounts for healthy functioning.

As it turns out, carbohydrates (or carbs) are the macronutrient our bodies need most.

Carbs often get a bad rap, especially with regard to weight gain. To be sure, some carbohydrates are better than others, but here are a few reasons we need carbohydrates to survive: carbs are the body's main source of fuel; they're easily converted into energy; carbs are important to intestinal health and waste elimination.

Carbs come in all shapes, sizes, and colors. You'll find them in both foods and beverages. Common sources of carbohydrates are fruits, vegetables, milk, nuts, and grains.

There are three types of carbohydrates: sugar, starch, and fiber. We'll talk about the importance of fiber in a moment.

According to the USDA's dietary guidelines, 45%–65% of calories should come from carbohydrates. This means for a 2000-calorie diet, between 900-1,300 of your calories should be carbohydrates.

For a diet healthy in carbohydrates, reach for fiber-rich fruits and vegetables. Choose whole grains that are rich in vitamins and minerals and naturally low in fat. And be smart with your dairy: choose low-fat milk, cheese, and yogurt, to name a few.

✚ WHAT'S FIBER?

We've all heard about fiber, but what in tarnation is it? Maybe you've heard the term roughage. And maybe you've heard that fiber can get you moving to the bathroom even after everything seems to have, well, stopped moving.

If you're up on your fiber facts, you know that the American Dietetic Association reports that most of us only get about <u>half</u> of the daily recommended 21–30 grams of fiber. C'mon, half? That's not even close.

What's so special about something that sounds only slightly more appetizing than plywood?

Fiber is a type of carbohydrate that the body can't digest. It's the structural part of plant foods that isn't broken down by our digestive system. You'll find fiber in many foods, including grains, vegetables, fruit, and legumes. Most of the fiber in fruits and vegetables is in the skin, so be sure not to peel it away. Navy beans and kidney beans are fiber superstars. When you're looking for fiber in bread, be sure to look for bread made with whole-grain flour. Also look for whole-wheat pasta.

What's fiber good for? Like I said, it's an excellent natural laxative when enjoyed with a large glass of water. That's important, especially as you get older because as we all know, constipation becomes more of an issue with age. High-fiber diets have also been shown to lower cholesterol, decrease the risk of colon cancer, and make us feel fuller faster, so high-fiber diets are a healthy way to trim a few pounds.

Make sure to give yourself an extra pat on the back when you find fiber on your nutrition label. And eat plenty of high-fiber food like fruits, vegetables, beans, and whole grains. These are the "good" carbohydrates—nutritious, filling, and relatively low in calories.

"The idea of a healthy diet is not to skip the mouth-watering foods and eat pinecones and peach pits instead."

✚ MIGHTY, MIGHTY PROTEIN

Protein will be our last stop on the food label. When it comes to maintaining muscle, organs, connective tissue, skin, bones, teeth, blood—and even your DNA!—protein is your source.

There's a protein in your blood call antibodies (although it should be called pro-bodies for all its good work) that helps the body's immune system to fight bacteria and other toxins. Protein is also found in your body's messengers: hormones.

Eating too little protein isn't healthy, but neither is eating too much. Healthy diet guidelines say that 10% -30% of your diet should be protein. You'll find it in the usual places like lean red meat, poultry, fish, cheese, and milk. But some lesser-known protein powerhouses are nuts, beans, and tofu.

✚ CHOOSING HIGH-QUALITY FOODS

All this talk of protein has put me in the mood to fire up the grill and have a burger. Not only does that sound tasty, it's a delicious opportunity to talk about the quality of the foods we choose, and the consequences of those choices.

I'd like to tell you a story about a serving size, and food quality, and the "little extras" we sometimes add to our entrees. Now stay with me here folks, because sometimes my stories take the scenic route, but they'll arrive at their destination eventually.

I'm guessing many of you either knew or still know the pleasure of cutting a lawn. It's a fact that if you don't have good fuel in your lawnmower—if there are impurities like water in the gasoline—the lawnmower will run poorly, if at all.

The same goes for the fuel we put in us. If the ground beef we chose for our hamburger is lean, say 95% lean and 5% fat, it's very good fuel and we'll run well on it. If, on the other hand, we buy the cheapest, fattiest ground beef for our hamburger, that's poor fuel and our bodies' performance will suffer.

I know it's difficult to buy healthy foods like lean ground beef when the fattier beef right next to it is cheaper. And the beef next to that is cheaper still. But the quality of the meat dramatically affects the calories and the nutritional value of what you eat.

And boy do things change again based on the condiments and extras we slap on the burger. Things like lettuce and tomato versus bacon and cheese make a world of difference.

Look at the Battle of the Burgers chart on the next page. For each of the burgers, look at the calories and the nutritional information that we've been talking about. It's an eye-opening

BATTLE OF THE BURGERS

You'll be shocked at how different the total calories and nutritional
values can be when you switch the type of meat, the quality
of meat, the "extras," and the bun.

Burger #1

4 oz. 80% lean ground beef
1 slice American cheese
2 pieces of pork bacon

1 tbsp mayonnaise
1 oz. sautéed onions
white hamburger bun

CALORIES	PROTEIN (DV 50g)	TOTAL FAT (DV 65g)	SAT. FAT (DV 20g)	CARBS (DV 300g)	FIBER (DV 25g)	SODIUM (DV 2,500mg)
685	41g (82%)	45g (82%)	15g (69%)	27g (9%)	2g (8%)	1208 mg (48%)

*Are you kidding me! Look at the calories and sodium.
Plus you've consumed 82% of your daily fat in one food item.*

Burger #2

4 oz. 90% lean ground beef
1 lettuce piece
1 tomato slice

1 oz. raw onion
2 packets mustard (2 tsp)
whole wheat bun

CALORIES	PROTEIN (DV 50g)	TOTAL FAT (DV 65g)	SAT. FAT (DV 20g)	CARBS (DV 300g)	FIBER (DV 25g)	SODIUM (DV 2,500mg)
350	32g (64%)	14g (22%)	5g (25%)	24g (8%)	4g (16%)	432 mg (17%)

*Much better! You cut your calories almost in half,
and your sodium by over a third.*

Burger #3

4 oz. ground turkey patty
1 lettuce piece
1 tomato slice

1 oz. avocado
whole wheat bun

CALORIES	PROTEIN (DV 50g)	TOTAL FAT (DV 65g)	SAT. FAT (DV 20g)	CARBS (DV 300g)	FIBER (DV 25g)	SODIUM (DV 2,500mg)
305	37g (74%)	9g (14%)	2g (10%)	22g (7%)	5g (20%)	221 mg (9%)

Ask yourself, is burger #1 really worth 68% more total fat?

demonstration of how our food choices add up, for better and for worse. If you're going to have a burger, make a good lean burger. And carefully choose the extras you put on it.

Bottom line: the idea of a healthy diet is not to skip the mouth-watering foods and eat pinecones and peach pits. The idea is to understand portion sizes, and to know the daily allowance of nutrition and calories that each portion brings to your plate. So when you're done cutting the lawn and you're hungry for a burger, you know exactly the right choices to make. See—I told you my stories arrive home, eventually.

And by the way, the same lesson goes for fruits and vegetables: not all of them are of equal quality, either. Shopping for fresh, nutritious fruits and vegetables is important. Unfortunately, one frustrating reality in America today is that in too many communities, these fresh choices aren't readily available. There is a name for this phenomenon: "food deserts."

"Remember the 8 X 8 rule: drink eight eight-ounce glasses of water daily."

The good news is that responsible retailers are beginning to address these deficits, and innovative thinkers are expanding farmer's markets, food co-ops, and community gardens, among other solutions. One of the greatest gifts that Dr. You

DR. YOU MEDICAL NOTE:

It takes the stomach approximately 15 to 20 minutes to tell the brain that you're full. Oftentimes, we will eat beyond being full because the news hasn't registered yet.

can give to yourself—as well as to your community—is to support and participate in the healthy food movement. Go forth and eat well!

✚ WATER: DRINK UP

Water is the fountain of life. About 60% of your body weight is water. Water carries nutrients to cells, flushes toxins from the body, and is instrumental to proper digestion. In short, you want to be a glass-half-full person in more ways than one.

A significant part of your healthy diet should be good old-fashioned water. Did you know that very few people actually drink enough of it? And it's free, too. That's right: good old tap water is perfectly okay.

Regardless of whether you choose water by the faucet or your favorite bottled brand, a great rule of thumb is the 8 x 8: eight glasses of water, eight ounces each, every day. Do not dismiss the 8 x 8 rule as something you don't need to bother with. Regardless of your size or your activity level, stay well hydrated. The exception to the 8 x 8 rule would be if your physician has restricted your daily intake of fluids due to a medical condition.

Among other things, water keeps you feeling full, which makes it a zero-calorie substitute for something significantly more calorie-dense. Furthermore, let's say you're feeling dizzy, struggling with fatigue or constipation, or experiencing frequent headaches. It could be dehydration. Water, water, water. Cheers!

✚ EAT SLOWLY

Here's a healthy eating tip that's very much out of line with the hustle and bustle of our culture and our times: go slowly, America. Heck, we coined the phrase "fast food." We don't eat slowly. We wolf down our food!

That is a problem. You see, it takes the stomach about 15 to 20 minutes to tell the brain "We're good; we're full." Oftentimes, you'll eat beyond the point of being full because the news that you're full hasn't registered yet.

Yes, I agree; that sounds strange. But it's true. It's called the satiety signal—satiety meaning being fed to the point of or beyond capacity.

Research shows again and again that when the same person slows down while eating, he or she consumes less food, and therefore fewer calories. That's because the stomach had time to get the message to the brain.

Try this at home. Finish eating dinner. Push away from the table satisfied, but not stuffed. Let's say you're still craving a little dessert. Just wait 15 or 20 minutes. Guess what? You probably won't be hungry for those extra bites after time passes.

Have you ever wondered why some waiters don't wait to rush the dessert cart to your table at the restaurant when the dinner plates have hardly been cleared? Suddenly you're surrounded by five-star service? Nah. They just may be trying to beat the satiety signal.

These are the golden years, right? I know you're busy, but don't rush through meals. In fact, don't rush through life. Slow down. Relax. Crazy as it may sound, light a candle. Think

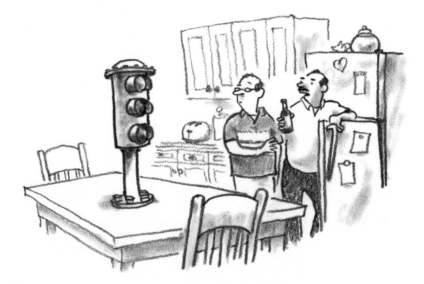

*"Loretta's hoping it will slow me
down when I eat."*

"dining" rather than "eating." Make dinner a social event. Bring the food out to the table in smaller courses, one by one. The extra time you take with your food will make a difference in less food consumed. *Bon appétit, mesdames et messieurs*!

✚ SUPPORT YOUR SPOUSE OR LOVED ONE

What if your new healthy diet is met with zero reaction or even a hostile response by your spouse or friends? They may consider it an inconvenience and try to ignore it, or declare that eating healthy is no big deal—despite the fact that you're working very, very hard at it.

> **"Unquestionably, it's best to embark on a change in diet as a pair—or as a household—but it doesn't always work out that way."**

Or, worse yet, what if the response is negative because "you're no fun to eat with"? You could also hear that your new diet is getting in the way of the two of you visiting your favorite greasy spoon, or that it's too expensive and a waste of time and money. You could be made to feel guilty because some meals will require special preparation to satisfy health needs or personal taste.

DR. YOU MEDICAL NOTE:

Support and make compromises for your loved one's diet change.

Unquestionably, it's best to embark on a change in diet as a pair—or as a household—but it doesn't always work out that way. Sometimes it takes months or years for your partner or family to see the light (or lite).

As we discussed at the opening of this chapter, your diet isn't a fad, it's a lifestyle change. It's going to take time for everyone. Keep the lines of communication open, knowing that the adjustment will likely create some tension, both emotionally and financially.

Dear Reader, the key is to support each other on this new venture. Take it slowly. Don't try to change everything in your diet at once. Make some compromises by occasionally going to the other's favorite restaurant; see if there are alternative menu choices that will work. Talk to the waitstaff or the cook about food ideas that are right for you—including not salting your food during preparation, serving salad dressing on the side, and not buttering your toast. You'll be surprised that more often than not, they're willing to find ways to keep you happy and healthier as a customer. After all, they want you coming back for years and years.

DR. YOU MEDICAL NOTE:

If you're overweight, lose 10% of your total weight and gain significant quality of life in return.

+ THE 10% RULE

Most overweight people can shed pounds and feel better by eating a healthier diet and becoming more active. What's more, most people need goals to motivate them; I'm especially that way. If you're overweight, here's an easy-to-grasp, easy-to-remember goal: lose 10% of your weight and gain significant quality of life in return.

Studies with people just like you and me have shown that a 10% decrease in body weight can have significant positive impacts on your health.[4] You can do 10%. I'm not saying it's easy, but I know a lot of people who have done it. They literally got sick and tired of carrying unhealthy weight. So they lost it. And it changed them, physically, mentally, and emotionally. This is doable, folks. And very, very worthwhile.

Don't fall into the trap of making excuses. I've heard them all. "I was born with bad genes." "It's a thyroid problem." "I just look at food and it sticks to my hips." Even if that were the case, we all can make adjustments to our diet that can be a life-changer. Remember the 10% rule. Decide today to eat healthier and trim 10% of your body weight. You will feel 100% better.

✚ TIPS THAT WORK FOR ME

- Instead of full-calorie, full-fat foods such as salad dressings, soups, and dairy, use lite versions.

- Eat your colors: make sure to include green, orange, and yellow fruits and vegetables. The antioxidants and other nutrients in these foods may help protect against developing certain types of cancer and other diseases.

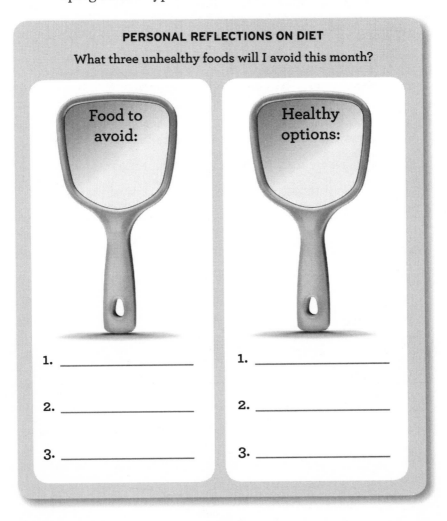

PERSONAL REFLECTIONS ON DIET

What three unhealthy foods will I avoid this month?

Food to avoid:

Healthy options:

1. _____

2. _____

3. _____

1. _____

2. _____

3. _____

- Nature's candy: eat fruit when craving sweets.

- The first three bites of food are always the best. Eat slowly, savor those bites.

- Supermarket's outside aisles: shop the outer ring of grocery stores. Typically the healthiest, least-processed foods are there.

- Eat less, more often, but be sure not to skip any meals. Sometimes five smaller meals is a better eating strategy than three larger ones.

- To save money, poke around the refrigerator and pantry before you shop so you don't double up on items that will go to waste.

- Find healthy food bargains. Often healthy foods are price-reduced for quick sale as they near their "sell by" date. Talk to your grocer. You could save 30–50%.

- Get a scale and know your weight for constant reinforcement and tracking your goals.

- Try something new, like tofu, for example. You'll be amazed. There are so many new healthy ways to prepare food—a whole new world awaits.

- Compare sodium in soups, breads, and frozen meals. Choose the lower numbers.

- Produce that's in season is usually on sale. Eat what's in season and save.

- Try Stevia and other natural zero-calorie sweeteners.

- Snack on sugar-free gum or hard candies between meals.

- Splurge a little: a small piece of dark chocolate or a cookie now and again isn't the end of the world.

- Food safety: It's reported that food poisoning by salmonella has increased by 10% in recent years. Wash your perishables under cold running water before eating them. Clean your countertops and cutting boards with soap and hot water. Beware of mayo-based dressings and salads left outdoors at summer events without proper refrigeration. Wash your hands. As I'm sure you've seen on the news, salmonella is a killer.

- Eat only at the table. No snacks at the computer station, in front of the TV, or in the car.

- When out to eat, bring home some of your meal in a doggie bag for tomorrow.

- Bruised produce can be a great bargain. Just cut out the bruise, and the high price.

- Fast food no more than two times a month.

- No eating after eight p.m.

- Use light cooking oils like canola and olive oil.

- Get a small four- or six-ounce container (think Tupperware®) to control the portion size of snacks.

- Brush (and floss) after meals. It signals your brain that you're finished eating—and dental health is linked to heart health.

DOCTOR'S ORDERS
HEALTHY DIET

R
X

- As Hippocrates said, "Let food be your medicine and your medicine be your food."

- A good rule of thumb: consume 2000 calories a day. (Consult with your doctor if you're on a special diet.)

- Eat a "colorful plate" with fruits and vegetables leading the way. See choosemyplate.gov.

- Read and compare food nutrition labels to achieve the best daily percentages and values. It's fun to find the foods that "win!"

- A good target number for your cholesterol is around 200 mg/dl, with LDL at around 130 mg/dl and HDL at around 60 mg/dl.

- Eat lean meats, lots of fiber from fruits, vegetables, and whole grains, and watch your cholesterol and sodium.

- Remember the 8 X 8: drink eight eight-ounce glasses of water daily.

- Slow down when eating. It takes your stomach 15 to 20 minutes to tell your brain that you're full.

- If you're overweight, losing 10% of your weight is proven to have immediate health benefits.

Dr. You

BATTLE OF THE BURGERS

Burger #1	CALORIES
4 oz. 80% lean ground beef	280
1 slice American cheese	94
2 pieces of pork bacon	85
1 tbsp mayonnaise	105
1 oz sautéed onions	35
White hamburger bun	115
Total	685

Burger #2	
4 oz. 90% lean ground beef	230
1 lettuce piece	5
1 tomato slice	5
1 oz raw onion	10
2 packet mustard (2 tsp)	5
whole wheat bun	95
Total	350

Burger #3	
4 oz. ground turkey patties	155
1 lettuce piece	5
1 tomato slice	5
1oz avocado	45
whole wheat bun	95
Total	305

*Calories are rounded to the nearest 5 and 10 digits
All nutritional information was obtained from the USDA Nutrient Data Laboratory
FDA's Food Guidance Compliance Regulatory Information /

BATTLE OF THE BURGERS

PROTEIN (G) (DV 50G)	TOTAL FAT (G) (DV 65G)	SAT. FAT (G) (DV 20G)	CARBS (G) (DV 300G)	FIBER (G) (DV 25G)	SODIUM (MG) (DV 2,500MG)
27 / (54%)	18 / (28%)	7 / (35%)	0 / (0%)	0 / (0%)	94 / (4%)
5 / (10%)	7 / (11%)	4 / (20%)	2 / (1%)	0 / (0%)	359 / (14%)
6 / (12%)	6 / (9%)	2 / (10%)	0 / (0%)	0 / (0%)	384 / (15%)
0 / (0%)	12 / (18%)	2 / (10%)	0 / (0%)	0 / (0%)	73 / (3%)
0 / (0%)	3 / (5%)	0 / (0%)	2 / (0%)	1 / (4%)	3 / (0%)
3 / (6%)	2 / (3%)	1 / (5%)	22 / (7%)	1 / (4%)	210 / (8%)
41 / (82%)	45 / (69%)	15 / (75%)	27 / (9%)	2 / (8%)	1208 / (48%)

29 / (58%)	12 / (18%)	5 / (25%)	0 / (0%)	0 / (0%)	85 / (3%)
0 / (0%)	0 / (0%)	0 / (0%)	1 / (0%)	0 / (0%)	7 / (0%)
0 / (0%)	0 / (0%)	0 / (0%)	1 / (0%)	0 / (0%)	1 / (0%)
0 / (0%)	0 / (0%)	0 / (0%)	3 / (1%)	1 / (4%)	81 / (3%)
0 / (0%)	0 / (0%)	0 / (0%)	1 / (0%)	0 / (0%)	114 / (5%)
3 / (6%)	2 / (3%)	0 / (0%)	18 / (6%)	3 / (12%)	144 / (6%)
32 / (64%)	14 / (22%)	5 / (25%)	24 / (8%)	4 / (16%)	432 / (17%)

33 / (66%)	3 / (5%)	1 / (5%)	0 / (0%)	0 / (0%)	67 / (3%)
0 / (0%)	0 / (0%)	0 / (0%)	1 / (0%)	0 / (0%)	7 / (0%)
0 / (0%)	0 / (0%)	0 / (0%)	1 / (0%)	0 / (0%)	1 / (0%)
1 / (2%)	4 / (6%)	1 / (5%)	2 / (0%)	2 / (8%)	2 / (0%)
3 / (6%)	2 / 3%)	0 / (0%)	18 / (6%)	3 / (12%)	144 / (6%)
37 / (74%)	9 / (14%)	2 / (10%)	22 / (7%)	5 / (20%)	221 / (9%)

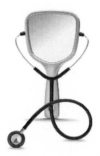

CHAPTER 4

BE ACTIVE

✚ BEING ACTIVE GIVES OUR LIVES PURPOSE

Dear Reader, I must say, this next topic is near and dear to my heart. This means you're about to embark on one of my favorite chapters. To say that I'm a big believer in being active is an understatement. My wife says I'm so active she needs a pair of wings to keep up. I tell her she does have wings—just like all the other angels. (When buttering up your spouse, don't hold back. When buttering up your bread, just use a dab the size of your thumb.)

> **"Being active is how you fulfill your purpose in life."**

To be clear, being active entails much more than running around in a sweatsuit flexing your muscles. Being active is how you fulfill your purpose in life. It's how you grow to become a "complete" person, actively sharing your talents with others.

It starts with setting goals. Fortunately, a residual benefit of having goals is it's great medicine; having goals and actively pursuing them staves off illness.

There are three ways to be active: physically active, mentally active, and socially active. By setting goals in each of these areas, life begins to fill with purpose, joy, and energy. Each type of activity is as important as the next, and each works in alignment with the next—like meshing gears. In this life, the body, mind, and soul all need to be stirred. Being active—getting your gears moving—makes life so much richer and fuller, as well as healthier. So let's set goals and let's get moving.

✚ OVERCOMING INERTIA

Let's begin by divulging the secret to being physically active. It's something that I'm confident every one of you can do. This secret doesn't require special shoes, or bulging muscles, or

DR. YOU MEDICAL NOTE:

There are three ways to be active: physically, mentally, and socially.

hardcore training. Ready? Drum roll please: the secret is you gotta move. You gotta move!

I know, I know. All my years of higher education should have taught me to use more refined, grammatically correct language. Forget grammar! You gotta move! You gotta WANT to move! Moving is life, plain and simple.

Our bodies crave movement—to burn calories, to get all the systems up and humming. So get up. If you're able and the weather is cooperating, get outdoors. Feel the sunshine on your face. Hear the birds and inhale the fresh air. Lift your grandchild to the sky. Walk briskly with your spouse, your partner, or a friend. If you can't get outside, stand up, turn on some music, and stretch out. Greet the wonderful gift of today by opening your body to it with movement.

Our bodies have more than 600 muscles.[1] We use approximately 225 of them just to take a step. It's amazing how these muscles work in harmony. Do you know why? Because they were made to move—in concert. When we move, our brain is engaged, the systems of our body are put on alert, our heart rate increases, muscles respond—all the way down to a cellular level.

DR. YOU MEDICAL NOTE:

By age 80, without an exercise regimen, we can lose roughly 44% of our muscle mass and 50% of our strength.

Wow. So much from one simple, beautiful movement.

Experts tell us that in our 40s, we lose 3%–8% of our muscle mass. And after age 50, the decline increases to 10%–20% per decade. That can add up to about a 44% percent loss in muscle mass by the time you reach 80. And that translates to roughly a 50% loss in strength.[2] Unless we do something about it, we're talking about some serious loss.

Enough about loss. Let's talk about gain. You're never too old to add muscle mass. There have been studies with seniors between the ages of 70 to 98 who have added upper- and lower-body weight training to their lives, netting whopping results—including significantly increased muscle strength, walking endurance, and walking speed. They reported that there were activities they couldn't do before weight training, but after 10 short weeks, they could accomplish. Some folks were resigned to a lifestyle severely limited by aging, but after strength training, reported a new lease on life.

"Your goal could be to win a bike race, or to play more actively with your grandkids, or to develop stronger arms and legs for getting out of chairs independently."

Let me give you an example of a gentleman I recently met who is an absolute inspiration. I'm going to call him the Sultan of Cycling. He's about to turn 70—a significant milestone indeed. So he set himself a goal: a cross-country relay race by bicycle. The Sultan and three other 70-somethings will each take turns cycling 20-minute stretches, from California all the way to the East Coast. Pedaling continuously as a relay team, it will take the four of them approximately seven days—and they won't be lollygagging; they want to set a new speed record for their age group. I find the Sultan of Cycling so inspiring because he shows us that we all need goals. It doesn't need to be a cross-country race; it could be crossing other personal boundaries that have held you back. Your goal could be to walk 15 minutes per day, three days a week. Your goal could be to play more actively with your grandkids, or to develop stronger arms and legs for getting out of chairs independently. You need to identify your goals, own them, and achieve them.

Why aren't we more physically active? There are a number of reasons, some more persuasive than others. One poor excuse is television. As we said earlier, seniors, on average, watch about seven hours of TV daily. In a way, that TV is plugged into you, sapping your energy. What a waste of vigor and life. Physical activity used to be an American hallmark. We have always been a pioneering bunch with an active spirit on a quest for a better way. Remember back a few pages when we talked about health

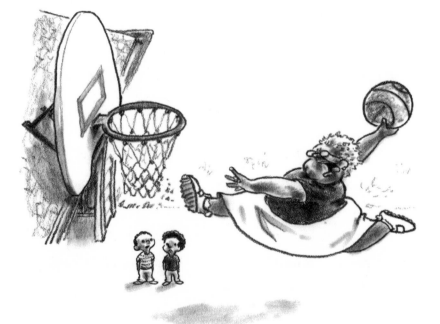

"Looks like Grammy has been using the ankle weights we got her."

being patriotic? Being active is a longstanding example of that. I realize that there is some worthwhile television programming, and having a few favorite programs or events to watch is fine, but a problem today is the availability of so darn many channels. You can't scroll through the TV menu without finding something fun to watch. But come on—it's literally a waste of life. Hit the Off button on the remote and the On button on life. Start by substituting one hour from the boob tube for a routine of stretching and physical exercise. You'll be amazed at how much better you feel in as little as five weeks. Plus, as we'll discuss later, there are a number of activities you can do while watching television that will make your body happy.

As much as anything, you just need to "get the ball rolling"—we've all heard that saying. Success begins with overcoming inertia, which isn't easy. The word inertia comes from the Latin word *iners*, meaning idle or lazy. But there's much more to it than that.

Newton used fundamentals of physics to tell us that a body at rest tends to stay at rest. (No, he wasn't talking about a body on the couch, but the same law pretty much applies.) You need to break inertia, or in other words, break the resistance that is keeping you motionless. Inertia is an exceptionally powerful force.

It takes tremendous quantities of mental and physical energy to get something that's motionless to move. I have heard it said that for a transatlantic flight, a jet can burn up to 50% of its fuel just getting off the ground and reaching cruising altitude.

Here's a situation you can probably relate to. Have you ever stood thigh-deep in a cool lake, seemingly stuck, unable to take the full body plunge? But once you dive in, the water feels fabulous and you wonder what held you up in the first place? That's inertia. The same goes for getting your routine of physical activity going. Once you've taken the plunge, it's wonderful. Because movement comes naturally.

What are your barriers to exercise? What inertia is holding you back, keeping you from getting out of your chair? Maybe physical activity wasn't a part of your upbringing. Maybe you

INERTIA IS HARD TO OVERCOME

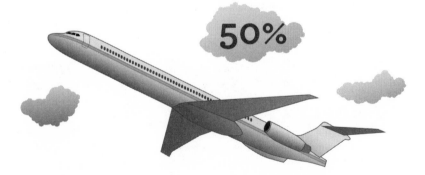

A jet can burn up to 50% of its fuel just getting off the ground and reaching cruising altitude.

think, It's too late for me. Maybe you think, I don't have the right workout outfit. Maybe you just don't like the idea of sweating (remember, sweat is one way your body rids itself of harmful toxins).

Let's address some of the major types of inertia—what I call the "Too Excuses"—that you must overcome to get your ball rolling. Thankfully, you're at an age where you don't have to worry about six-pack abs or perfect biceps or physical attributes that will win you a photo shoot for the cover of a fitness magazine. This is about reducing and eliminating the barriers between you and a more physically active life.

It might seem like a long way from here to there, but becoming that person is within reach. When you're done with this section, Dr. You will have some very achievable ideas, tips, and goals. I know you have the physical strength and the intestinal fortitude to get there. All you need is a simple plan to get you going, starting with eliminating a few of the biggest excuses we all encounter.

✚ "I'M IN TOO MUCH PAIN"

A very small percentage of you truly are in too much pain for physical activity. You're just getting by, day to day, and you don't want to hear any rah-rah speeches about silver linings and the indomitable human spirit. I understand that, respect that, and you have my deepest sympathies. Hopefully your doctor is doing everything medically possible to help you manage your pain.

But there are only a small percentage of you who suffer from such extreme, chronic, debilitating pain that you can't become more active. There are times when a doctor has to dispense unpopular advice—call it a dose of tough love. That isn't always immediately appreciated. As the doctor in the mirror, you know when a dose of reality is called for. Let's not hold onto unnecessary barriers when we don't have to. In consultation with your doctor, find the maximum activity level that your body will allow. You can do it.

It's time you found your will. Combine that with this bountiful chapter of practical, in-home and out-of-home activities, and you can arrive at a place you hardly dared dream possible. Such are the health benefits of a more active lifestyle.

To be sure, as increased activity becomes more integral to your weekly routine, you will encounter some sore, tired muscles and aggravated joints. You don't need to jump right on a regular dose of aspirin or acetaminophen (Tylenol®). Some discomfort is natural and to be expected; it's your body sending you a message that it's back in the game. Ice and heat, massage, baths, and stretching are great non-pharmaceutical pain relievers. Of course, always consult your doctor if your pain persists. And if you need an <u>occasional</u> pain reliever, use it carefully.

For soreness and pain, the question eventually comes around to, "what's better: ice or heat?" Ice is a great place to start, especially if the pain is caused by overuse or a recent injury and you need to decrease swelling around the affected area right after exercise. Be sure to always ice after your activity, but never before. If the pain is less acute and is more of an everyday soreness, heat treatments can be just the ticket. Heat will dilate blood vessels in the muscle, and stimulate the flow of blood rich in oxygen and healthy nutrients to help repair damaged tissue. Heat also facilitates stretching of muscles and tissue, so it can be used before the activity.

Bottom line on pain: for a very small percentage of older adults, your pain is too great; therefore physical activity is not recommended. For the others, don't accept pain as a lifelong barrier to physical activity. Here's why: pain begets pain. Said another way, pain can be the starting point in a chain of events that can lead to more pain and ever worsening health. Visualize pain as a run of tipping dominoes where pain leads to being sedentary, which leads to being unhealthy, which leads to further illness—and down the line it goes.

Or visualize something quite the opposite: being active leads to being healthy, which leads to strength, which leads to being active, which leads to a better quality of life. Imagine how your healthy domino run can produce a more joyful, spectacular life.

Speaking of joyfully spectacular—not to mention dominoes—if you have a spare moment, get a move on over to your computer and view one of coolest domino runs you've ever seen. Google "youtube 5300 homemade dominos." My hope is it will help you remember that tipping one domino in the right direction can lead to amazing things.

+ "IT'S TOO LATE FOR ME"

Perhaps the most common excuse for not being physically active is your belief that too many years of bad habits can't be undone. Do you consider yourself past the point of no return? Too overweight? Too ill? Too far gone? If you do, listen to me. There's no such thing.

As the Chief of Medical Affairs for UnitedHealth Group, I have the privilege of collaborating with some of the finest physicians, hospitals, and health care professionals in the world—including care managers who work every day on the front lines of health. These nurses and other health professionals have witnessed and helped bring about some truly amazing health turnarounds in the day-to-day lives of the patients they serve.

I get to see firsthand what's working in the field of elder health, and how people are finding newfound vitality and joy in life even after years of quite the opposite. From complex studies to everyday stories, the proof is there. The path to a better life, thanks to all this learning, and the wise assistance of my colleagues, is here in the pages you hold in your hands. Time and time again, we've seen examples of people thinking the joy and health in their life was all but gone, only to have turned it around, slowly, but surely. And that is the secret: a slow pace is better than no pace. (Remember: a penny at a time.)

But first you have to believe. How does the 90/10 principle go again? I'm paraphrasing, but it's something like: 10% of life is what happens to you. The other 90% is how you deal with it. Whatever your situation might be, from pretty good to awfully bad, take the 90% that you can control and decide it's not too late to make things better. Not even close to too late. Open the door and allow greatness to enter into your life.

✚ "IT'S TOO EXPENSIVE TO JOIN A GYM"

I agree that health club memberships can sometimes be pricey for many of our budgets. But if you have the money, there is no better long-term investment you can make for the dollar. Forget about stocks and bonds and gold futures—invest in your golden future.

For folks who don't have the disposable income to spend on a health club membership, I'm going to make it very easy to turn your home into a wonderful exercise facility. And just think: at your gym there will be no hassles finding a parking spot. No waiting in line to exercise. And no keeping up with the Joneses when it comes to having a perfect outfit for your workout. (What color goes best with sweat, anyhow?)

It's pretty easy to make your home an exercise-friendly environment. Start by looking at how your furniture is arranged. If you're able, move a few small pieces out of the way, clearing a little space for you to do your thing whenever you want. As you'll see, you don't need much space for stretching and calisthenics such as sit-ups, modified push-ups, and jumping jacks. As we'll talk about very soon, even your favorite chair can be turned into an excellent workout aid.

"Your heart is in the right place as you busily provide for others, but your well-placed heart will suffer from lack of exercise."

Purchase an exercise mat for the floor that can be easily rolled up and stored. Get a few inexpensive, light hand weights (or just use a water bottle or cans of soup), a rubber exercise band for strength and flexibility work, and if possible, an exercise bike or treadmill for those days when you can't get outside for your cardiovascular exercise. You can find some great deals on used equipment if you're willing to look. And think about it: is there really a better investment you could make than an investment in you?

Making your home exercise-friendly doesn't take much, so don't make it a big deal. The point is to do something—big or small. And discover you'll have fun doing so.

> ### DON'T LET THE "TOO EXCUSES" KEEP YOU FROM EXERCISING
>
> - I'm in too much pain
> - It's too late for me
> - It's too expensive to join a gym
> - I'm too busy
> - It's too complicated
> - I'm too afraid of falling or injuring myself
> - It's too hot, it's too cold, or it's just too something

✚ "I'M TOO BUSY"

Make time for yourself, okay? I don't know how to say it any more clearly. You're no good to anyone if you become incapacitated by illness. Yes, your heart is in the right place as you busily provide for others, take care of the house, work overtime, become a caregiver for your grandchildren, and the like, but your well-placed heart will suffer from lack of exercise. As will the rest of your body.

Folks, when you think of exercise, you need to think of activity above and beyond your usual daily routine. Start with simple goals like elevating your heart rate for 15 to 30 minutes per day, most days of the week, because that will help your heart and cardiovascular system function more effectively. And incorporate weight-bearing exercises like walking, climbing stairs, and weight training to build strong bones and keep muscles toned so you can perform your everyday activities. Yes, being busy is good, but don't fool yourself that it's the same as exercise.

If there's time for everyone else, there's time for you. Dr. You has to find a way to work exercise into the daily routine. Please, make yourself a priority.

✚ "IT'S TOO COMPLICATED"

Getting started with a routine of physical activity, as we talked about earlier, is challenging in more ways than one. Maybe you hail from a nonathletic background and don't know what exercises to do, or how to perform them. Or you're afraid of falling or injuring yourself. Certainly, if you have any questions or concerns about the physical activity you're about to add to your life, check with your primary physician or health professional first. But I'll be giving you plenty of good, simple ideas to chose from.

Of all the reasons I hear about why someone is not engaged in physical activity, one of the most credible is, "I don't have the foggiest idea where to start." For example, how far should I walk? How much weight should I lift? How many repetitions? How do I improve my balance?

As I myself have aged, I continue to be taught by the example and expertise of my still very physically active and exercise-dedicated mother, as well as colleagues who are experts in the field of senior fitness. I've come by a wealth of information on how to get started. So get ready to learn a number of simple, very doable exercises that will make a difference in your day, and in your life.

"Stretching is the simple process of aligning mind, body, and spirit."

I want you to start by thinking positive. That is the key to unlocking so much progress. So what if you have two left feet, flabby arms, and get winded looking at stairs. Shoot, I've heard them all. Let's start small. We'll get it going—don't sweat it. Wait, let me rephrase. Let's sweat it during and after the exercise, but not before.

Before you start, especially if you've been inactive for a long period of time, it's always wise to consult with your primary care physician. You can also evaluate potential risk by using the EASY tool (Exercise And Screening for You) found online at www.easyforyou.info.

Our motto for this chapter, as well as this book: keep it simple and start it easy. Begin with the little things. Now a few of you may be saying to yourself, "Think small? I'm not going to get very far with that philosophy. I need a bigger challenge."

Let me tell you a story about Michael Jordan. Chances are you've heard of the man who many call the greatest basketball player of all time. He won six NBA championships, and was a five-time NBA Most Valuable Player. What was a major factor in his success, his durability, his leaping ability, and his long playing career? Physically, he focused on the little things that didn't draw a lot of attention. Not bulging arms covered in muscles and tattoos, or a huge button-popping chest. He worked on his wrists, forearms, fingers, ankles, calves, feet, and balance. Little things. Will you be able to leap like Michael Jordon after this chapter? Maybe, in your sleep. My point is, he proves that working on the little things can add up to big things. As you make progress, you can add incrementally more to your exercise routine—in fact you should, because progress is extremely motivating. But start small and practical, because if it's not practical, what good is it, and what fun is it?

Let's revisit the joy of moving. Start by moving your arm. Feel it slip through space as the thousands of nerve endings in your skin sing to your brain that your arm is in motion. Track your movement with your eyes (that is when you're done reading these sentences) as you now move both arms, letting your fingers meet over your head before they come back to your sides. Imagine a return to childhood. Making snow angels—or for you luckier ones, making beach angels. Are you doing it? If this activity sounds silly, you know what? You're too tight. You have to loosen up!

"The solid foundation of exercise, both literally and figuratively, is balance."

✚ SIX BUTTERFLIES SIPPING COCOA

Let's follow up those simple movements by concentrating on the foundation of your exercise routine. There are four parts, and the way I remember them is with this funny little phrase: Six Butterflies Sipping Cocoa.

Notice the first letters of each word in my odd little sentence? The S, B, S and C are capitalized so you'll remember them. The S is for stretching. The B is for balance. The next S is for strength. And the C is for cardio, or cardiovascular exercise. Six Butterflies Sipping Cocoa. Stretching, Balance, Strength, Cardio. Got it?

If everyday you wake up and attend to your Six Butterflies Sipping Cocoa, you're going to be in great shape—in more ways than one. Again, keep it simple, and keep it doable.

SIX BUTTERFLIES SIPPING COCOA (SBSC)

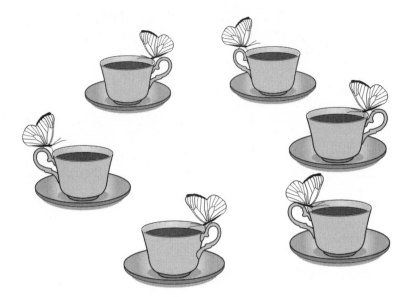

Stretching, balance, strength training, and cardio fitness are four areas crucial to healthy aging. That's how Dr. You slowly but surely takes control of the physical fitness piece of your health.

✚ STRETCHING

Of course, before exercise begins, it's time to stretch. In fact, stretching is how I recommend you start every day. Think of yourself as a storefront preparing to be opened in the morning. You wake up, unlock your doors, flip on your lights, sweep out the cobwebs, roll out your awning, and you're ready to

DR. YOU MEDICAL NOTE:

Four areas critical to healthy aging: stretching, balance, strength training, and cardio fitness.

greet the day. This is what stretching does for the systems of your body. It feels so good when muscles awaken, blood flows, joints unlock, and your mind opens to engage with every movement. This simple process of aligning mind, body and spirit—getting them all in tune—is the ideal way to get ready for the business of the day.

Speaking of business, there is one purchase I strongly suggest you make as you prepare for physical activity. Buy a good pair of athletic shoes. They shouldn't cost you more than $75. Make sure they have ample arch support, fit correctly, and are well-cushioned. Heck, your first stretch can be to lean over and tie those new laces.

Stretching is essential to keeping your body as flexible and limber as can be so you can move with grace, preventing injury. A physical therapist friend of mine is fond of saying "motion is lotion." What he's teaching us is that moving lubricates joints and muscles so the body is freer to make the next movement.

Your stretching can be as simple or elaborate as you like—just be sure to make time for it. I suggest you go online and find the stretches that are best for your particular needs. That could mean Googling anything from "stretches for a sore back" to "stretching before biking" to "best morning stretches." You'll have to stretch your imagination to think of all the possibilities.

✚ BALANCE

The solid foundation of exercise, both literally and figuratively, is balance. Balance involves an intricate system of communication between your inner ear, eyes, muscles, joints, and brain. As we age, our ability to maintain balance often deteriorates and this can lead to falls. Some of the factors contributing to impaired balance can be poor posture, weight gain, weakened muscles, and low blood pressure.

Poor balance can also be a side effect of your medications or an unintended interaction of drugs that you're taking. Don't dismiss poor balance and the subsequent falls as mere embarrassments, inconsequential to health. As you'll see in Chapter 9, falls are the leading cause of debilitating injury among the elderly and a serious risk factor for premature death. So let's work hard on preventing them.

See a few of my favorite balance exercises coming up. And be sure to Google "balance exercises" for links to many more, including helpful videos. Remember to always keep your eyes open when performing balance exercises. And have a water bottle with you to stay fully hydrated as you go.

SIT TO STAND

1. Sit in the center of a sturdy chair. Chest lifted. Feet hip-distance apart on the floor.
2. Look forward, lean forward and come to a standing position. (You can use the chair's hand rests if you need to.)
3. Carefully return to the sitting position.

Do this exercise ten times. Repeat for three sets.

SIDE LEG RAISES

1. Standing tall, directly behind the chair, gently grasp the top of the chair.
2. Feet slightly apart.
3. Slowly lift your right leg six to ten inches out to the side, keeping hips level, with foot flexed, toe up, heel down.
4. Return your foot to the floor, and repeat same action with the other leg.

Do this exercise eight times for each leg. Repeat for two sets.

As your balance improves, you may want to take your hand off the chair, but keep it close should you lose your balance. Remember, safety first.

TAPPING THE BOOK

1. Put a medium-thickness book (perhaps a hardcover novel) on the floor at the side of your chair.

2. Stand at the side of the chair just behind the book.

3. Gently grasp the back of the chair with the hand nearest the chair.

4. Lift the outside leg and gently tap the book with your toe, then switch to the other leg.

5. Continue to alternate legs for 20 toe taps for each.

As with our previous exercise, when your balance improves, you may want to take your hand off the chair, but keep it close should you lose your balance.

✚ STRENGTH

Strength training builds lean muscle tissue that boosts your metabolism. Translation: you will burn calories while you're working out, and long after you're done. Nice bonus!

TWO GREAT ONLINE RESOURCES FOR EXERCISING

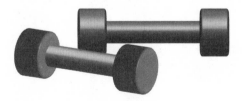

www.nia.nih.gov (click on Go4life)
www.eldergym.com

DR. YOU MEDICAL NOTE:

Elevate your heart rate for 15 to 30 minutes per day, most days of the week, and your heart and cardiovascular system will function more effectively.

Don't forget the important medical fact we discussed earlier: after age 50, muscle mass declines by 10%–20% per decade, and strength will decline right along with it.

But there is good news. Strength exercises can build overall strength and bone strength, increase everyday mobility, and burn fat. And strength is one of the keys to staying independent. If you're not strong, you can't squeeze the most out of anything, let alone life.

Before you engage in strength training—or any exercise—be sure to warm up with a stretching routine to help reduce the possibility of aches, pains, or injury. To find age-appropriate strength exercises, go to your bookstore, library, or online. A place to start is: www.nia.nih.gov (click on Go4life) or see great exercise ideas brought to life in short, helpful videos at www.eldergym.com.

✚ CARDIO

Elevating your heart rate shouldn't only happen when you're in the car snarled in traffic. We've talked about what a wonderful pump your heart is and how it provides blood flow through a miraculously vast circulatory system about the size of 20 trips across America. It literally is a matter of life or death to keep your heart as healthy as can be.

Cardiovascular exercise is a way to a healthier heart. Experts in the field say nearly all older adults can participate in moderate cardiovascular exercise such as a brisk walk for 30 minutes a day, most days of the week. But as we learned earlier, 44% of adults 65-plus are considered "inactive," meaning they engage in less than ten minutes of moderate or vigorous activity weekly. Come on; we can all do better.

"Elevating your heart rate shouldn't only happen when you're in the car snarled in a traffic jam."

If it's been a while since you've exercised, remember to build up slowly and gradually. As I've told you since page one, the way to feel like a million bucks is a penny at a time. You can start with as little as five or ten minutes each session. It's amazing how your endurance (and confidence) will build over time.

A few of my favorite moderate cardiovascular exercises include brisk walking, biking or stationary bike, chasing my grandchildren, sightseeing, dancing, swimming, and tai chi. For those you looking for more vigorous exercise, I like competitive cycling, jogging, and cross-country skiing. Try them all!

✚ MOM'S FIVE-MINUTE CHAIR WORKOUT

Before we move on, I'd like to share a few exercises that are near and dear to my heart. This routine comes from my mother, a nurse and exercise enthusiast. It can be done sitting in your favorite chair, watching the news on TV. If nothing else, I guarantee the news will get better.

NECK EXERCISES

1. Right ear to shoulder, back to center, left ear to shoulder. Repeat for five touches.
2. Turn head to right, back to center, turn head to left. Repeat five times.

SHOULDER EXERCISES

1. Rotate both shoulders toward back, with elbows making a small clockwise circle. Repeat five times.
2. Rotate both shoulders toward the front, with elbows making a small counterclockwise circle. Repeat five times.

FINGER EXERCISES

1. Open and close hands ten times, making a fist.
2. Then touch thumb to each finger, beginning with little finger, then ring, them middle, then index. Both hands, ten times.

ARM EXERCISES

1. Push right arm up with palm facing up. Simultaneously push left arm down with palm facing down. Hold each for count of four. Repeat ten times.

2. Put left palm in your right palm. Use your right arm to curl your left hand to your chest, providing some resistance from your left hand. Repeat ten times. Change hands, and repeat with the left arm.

ABDOMINAL EXERCISES

1. With arm bent waist-high, twist upper body to the right, back to center, then to left. Repeat ten times.

LEG EXERCISES

1. Raise right leg with toes pointing upward, hold and lower. Repeat ten times. Switch to left leg and repeat.

2. With feet on the floor, raise toes off the floor, then put them back down. Repeat ten times.

3. Repeat, this time raising heels off the floor and back down.

4. Curl right leg under the chair, and return foot to the floor. Repeat ten times.

5. Curl left leg under chair, and return foot to the floor. Repeat ten times.

6. With feet shoulder-width apart, rise slowly out of the chair ten times, with or without the use of armrests as your strength dictates.

✚ ROSARY AEROBICS

Here's one last all-time favorite exercises before we move on. I love it because it shows that barriers between you and physical activity can often times be overcome. This time with the help of prayer.

Rosary aerobics came from a friend's grandmother who lived to be over 100. Every morning she'd get out of bed and pray the rosary. She did the same thing before bedtime, too. But rather than sitting idle while saying her Hail Marys, she'd be up on her feet, moving around her bedroom. When she got through ten beads (known as a decade) she'd switch hands, which were busy making small clockwise and counterclockwise circles while holding the rosary (change direction after each Hail Mary). That's what she called rosary aerobics. Who knew that exercise could be so spiritual!

✚ BE A DYNAMO; EXERCISE WITH A GROUP

For those who can get out and find affordable exercise classes, great. A little peer pressure can be exactly what your body needs. Let me elaborate.

When exercising with others, there is a group dynamic that causes you to see what's possible, and reach for a higher level of performance. A person naturally wants to keep up (within your abilities) and stay with the group. This can be the motivation necessary to find your true potential (which may have gotten a little dusty and rusty) versus your perceived potential.

It can be as simple as exercising with your spouse, partner, or friend. You can motivate each other and, at the very least, keep each other honest about sticking to your routine at the appointed time.

Or, in other cases, your exercise group might be notably wider-reaching. Take, for example, Oklahoma City. The city is on track to collectively lose one million pounds by the end of 2011. The mayor—40 pounds overweight himself—presented a

CAN THE "FAST FOOD CAPITAL OF AMERICA" LOSE ONE MILLION POUNDS?

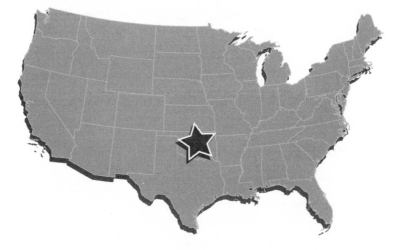

The power of group exercise.
See www.thiscityisgoingonadiet.com.

challenge to his city (dubbed the "Fast Food Capital of America" by *Fortune* magazine) when he learned that one in four citizens of Oklahoma County were obese, and one in three got virtually no exercise.

Healthier eating awareness, more walkable and bike-friendly streets, group walking, hiking, running events—and a group goal of shedding a million pounds—have helped the city make tremendously healthy strides. (See www.thiscityisgoingonadiet.com.) Louisville and Seattle have similar citywide programs in place.

TIPS TO HELP YOU STICK WITH YOUR ROUTINE

- Start slowly
- Work out with your loved one or a friend
- Vary your workout routine
- Put achievable end-of-the-month goals on the calendar
- Celebrate milestones and stick-to-itiveness by treating yourself to a monthly reward like a healthy meal out, a new article of clothing, a night at the movies, etc.
- Make it fun. Forget "no pain, no gain"

How do you join or start a group program? Check with your community center and places of worship to see what kind of exercise programs they might offer. If they don't have anything, don't stop there. Be a leader and get something started: walking clubs, a biking group, bowling teams, or group dance lessons once per week. Group exercise can be life-changing because you'll discover it provides strength in more ways than one.

As I mentioned earlier, if you can afford it, joining a health club is another fantastic option. Here you will find great instructors who can be motivating coaches to help you find your true potential. They can inform Dr. You when to taper back on your workout, and when to push forward. Again, it's always important to discuss your exercise routine with your doctor or health professional because they need to be in the loop on any sizable changes in your lifestyle. Chances are, they will be very proud and supportive of your new activities, but don't leave them out.

Sometimes just being in a health club setting and seeing other people engaging their bodies can be your inspiration. Better yet, finding age-appropriate classes can be both physically and socially beneficial. If you are able to get out and participate a few days per week in more organized exercise, I recommend classes such as tai chi, yoga, and water aerobics. Other actives such as riding a stationary bike, swimming, and high-repetition/low-weight strength training are also terrific.

✚ EXERCISE IS MEDICINE

Do a body inventory. Where do you ache, hurt, or suffer from stiffness? What are the areas of chronic pain? Now, what can you do about it? Just grin and bear it? Or take a pill for your every ill? Not so fast. There are many non-pharmaceutical remedies for body pains. And the one that doctors recommend most is exercise.

I know firsthand the challenges that come with aging. My motto is, "Don't take pain sitting down!" Get going and fight back with exercise. From our stiff necks to the burning plantar fasciitis in our feet, what's your Achilles' heel? More times than not, you can begin to alleviate, and in some cases eventually eliminate, your aches and pains by strengthening your body.

Everything about your body is interconnected, so an exercise that's good for, say, shoulders, is also good for your legs. How? Well if your shoulders are strong, then it's easier to get out of a chair and walk, which in turn strengthens leg muscles. Taking that a little further, moving those legs helps keep stiffness out of joints, and that brightens your disposition and lifts your spirits. Holy Toledo! Look what one simple shoulder exercise can do.

✚ BE ACTIVE MENTALLY

Let me remind you again that health is not the absence of pain or disease; it's a sense of mental, physical, and spiritual well-being. Being mentally active is critical to your health, now more than ever before. Please, dear Reader, keep your mind active by never losing your sense of curiosity.

DR. YOU MEDICAL NOTE:

Don't lose your sense of curiosity, because being active mentally is essential to your good health.

The word curiosity comes from the Latin *curiosus* meaning to be diligent and careful, and is akin to *cura*, which means care. So curiosity really is a type of care.

As for me, there isn't enough time in the day to read everything I want to read, talk to all the wise people I wish to speak to, and ponder all the mysteries of life knotted before me. That's okay. It gives me something to do tomorrow. Curiosity truly is a lifelong friend.

My curiosity with the wonders of the human body led me to medical school and becoming a doctor. And my curiosity with larger-scale health issues led me to being the commissioner of Public Health for the District of Columbia, my work with UnitedHealth Group, and the writing of this book. In between, I am an avid photographer and cyclist, as well as a jazz drummer. The pursuit of knowledge and excellence in these areas has kept me mentally fit, mentally young, and mentally strong. And I'm hoping the same can be said for you.

If you're retired, don't let your brain retire, too. Keep it working. Read newspapers, magazines, and books. Surf the Internet for information and answers, not only on your health, but pertaining to your interests. This is an amazing time we live

DR. YOU MEDICAL NOTE:

If you're retired, don't let your brain retire, too.

in, with unprecedented access to information right at your fingertips thanks to the World Wide Web.

Take up a new hobby. You can take a class, or if that's not realistic, you can learn a great deal about your interests online. If you don't have a home computer, go to your neighborhood library. They will greet you with a brass band. Say, for example, you're interested in keeping tropical fish in a saltwater aquarium. Great. The librarian will be all too happy to help you get comfortable working online, and will help you find books on the subject to bring home, too.

There are daily habits that help you stay active mentally. Wrestle with brainteasers, Sudoku, crossword puzzles, and the like. Maybe you're no good at them—perfect! That means you'll be learning something new, and research suggests that new learning takes us off autopilot, allowing the brain to form new neurological pathways, even stimulating the production of entirely new brain cells. When the brain isn't challenged, it atrophies, which can lead to dementia, Alzheimer's, and other brain diseases. Those are but a few very real reasons to keep your mind nimble and innovative.

Turn off the TV. Challenge yourself. Walk a new route around the block. Read or listen to an opinion that conflicts

DR. YOU MEDICAL NOTE:

Research suggests that new learning takes us off autopilot, allowing the brain to form new neurological pathways—even stimulating the production of entirely new brain cells.

with your own. Don't become stunted by certainty and habit. I've read that to decide too quickly is to kill off all possibilities but one. Keep an open and curious mind.

Chances are your improved mental health will go hand in hand with your improved physical health.

Make a promise to yourself to reach for your mental stretch zone. Don't get mentally flabby by refusing to move out of your comfort zone. And don't spend days on end in your mental stress zone where challenges are overwhelming. Your mental stretch zone is a wonderful place where you're actively seeking new information and experiences. You'll find that stretching is as beneficial for the mind as it is for the body.

You surely know the saying "you learn something new every day." Well, have you? C'mon, try it—on your own, with loved ones, or with an extended group. Find a new board game or dice game. (Did you know that dice are the oldest and most universal game pieces, and were likely first made with knucklebones? If not, chalk up a new thing learned.) Learn a new game of cards or how to play bridge (just Google "How to play bridge"). See a live performance such as a play or concert, or just let your mind ponder the endless beauty of nature. These are the years where you actually have some time for yourself—a sort of second childhood—to learn new things.

SEE ONE, DO ONE, TEACH ONE

A principle from medicine suggesting that seeing and doing lead to mastery, and with mastery comes the responsibility of teaching

---

If you're lucky enough to have grandchildren or great-grandchildren, teach them something that you know. In medicine there's a principle known as See One, Do One, Teach One. This means that seeing and doing lead to mastery, and with mastery comes the responsibility of teaching.

Undoubtedly, there's something you're fantastic at. Don't hoard it. Get off the couch and teach. When you do, you'll find another truism as a result: teaching is learning. And you will be creating intergenerational connections. Hopefully someday your grandchild will be a grandparent, passing down that teaching to the next generation of grandchildren. Wow, I'm getting mentally pumped up just thinking about all this.

Your brain is a marvelously complex, high-maintenance organ. It consumes an estimated 20% of your daily energy. It needs to be kept active to remain healthy. Which brings us full

DR. YOU MEDICAL NOTE:

Relationships, both intimate and platonic, are critical to our good health.

circle, back to curiosity, and how that trait plays a critical role in the quality and the longevity of your life. Curiosity didn't kill the cat, dear Reader. Curiosity is why the cat has nine lives.

✚ BE ACTIVE SOCIALLY

Because humans are social animals, it's only natural that we interact with one another. Relationships, both intimate and platonic, are critical to our good health.

But what about those who are shy or introverted or have lost their confidence? Or those who have lost a spouse and outlived friends and relatives and just "want to be left alone"? Please—being social doesn't mean you have to be the straw that stirs the drink, but it's unnatural and unhealthy to withdraw from society. Social isolation, closing doors behind you, shuttering your home and yourself from others can make you ill, and can lead to premature death.

So let's talk about how to be active socially because it's darn important to healthy aging. The way I see it, being socially active has two components: you can be publicly active and you can be emotionally active. For many of us, being emotionally active includes intimacy and sexuality. Let's look at these concepts one at a time.

A great place to be publicly active and connect with others is your place of worship. It starts with a nod, a wave, and a smile. A simple "good morning" or "beautiful day" isn't asking too much. Maybe there's coffee and cookies once a month—partake. There might be opportunities to help out and be active in your church or synagogue, mosque or temple. Unquestionably, there are some very nice people who would welcome your increased participation. Chances are they have some pretty cool stories to share, and so do you.

Another way, believe it or not, to become more socially active is shopping (sorry, guys). While shopping, there are numerous opportunities to meet, mingle, and talk with others—as well as workers. The grocery store, your favorite retail store, and the mall can be great places for fun, quick conversation.

Part-time jobs or volunteering are also super-healthy ways to get more out of life. These activities can do wonders for your mental health, too. And don't forget about fraternal organizations, civic associations, neighborhood groups, community clubs, and events. These types of social activities nourish us in a way that food cannot.

Being publicly active also means leveraging your "gray power." You've heard of the green movement and green power?

I'm talking about the gray movement. Folks, this is a very important and often overlooked aspect of getting older: you have the power to change things for the better for an aging America. Remember, we're all in this together.

Just take the 65-plus population, for example; it's the fastest-growing group in the country—increasing by about 1.5 million empowered people a year. The spending power of the 50-plus demographic is about three trillion dollars—up 45% in the past ten years.[3] What's more, seniors represent almost 20% of the presidential votes cast.[4] According to CNN, the senior vote represented 23% of all votes cast in the 2010 mid-term elections.[5] That's gray power.

News flash! You're part of a financial and political powerhouse. Create your own community caucus, or join groups that already exist. Use your political might to shape legislation that affects you, both on a national scale and at the grassroots community level. This can include everything from more affordable prescription drugs to lower costs for healthy food to better public transportation. At a community level, it could be adding or enhancing area walking paths, funding for community center programs, and better-lit neighborhoods for safer living conditions.

Don't sit back and complain—stand up and complain! Contact your district, state, and federal representatives. They work for you. Tell those whippersnappers (respectfully) to stop cutting senior services, and to start fighting for them. Or you'll vote them out. "Do not go gentle into that good night," as Dylan Thomas wrote.

Even if you don't use many senior services now, you may need them later. Remember, as we age we have to stick together because we're in this together. The goal is to create healthier communities.

"Leverage your 'gray power.' You're part of a financial and political powerhouse!"

To find your representatives, go to www.usa.gov. Don't stop there. Write letters to the editor of your paper. Get involved in local politics. Know what's happening with senior policy on a national level. Stand up for yourself and your peers. That's being socially active, and it is good.

✚ EMOTIONALLY ACTIVE

Don't shut down emotionally. Yes, relationships can be difficult—especially long-term relationships with their trials and tribulations. It can be easy to pull away from your spouse or partner and reside, in so many words, in your half of the home.

Emotional intimacy is about sharing. It's about verbal and non-verbal communication that says, "I care." Ultimately it's about trust.

Inevitably, aging will create some significant challenges; shore up the weak spots in your relationship that time has made thin. Talk to each other. Trust each other. Remember, two is better than one.

I want to give you a challenge: dare to share. You know what? It takes big-time courage to share. Get close. Be a team. The time is now.

Perhaps you're a person who by choice or by circumstance lives alone. Well guess what? This conversation applies to you, too. In the end, we all need people, and are better with people in our lives—even if we don't happen to share the same home. Later in the book, we'll talk about how family and friends can help make a safety net of relationships that we'll need inevitably. So everyone, take part in the following personal inventory with the goal of connecting better emotionally with others.

I want to respectfully ask that you be someone that another person *wants* to be close to. Think about your mood and disposition. I know some of you are suffering with chronic illnesses that make it difficult to think beyond your discomfort, but you must. If you're taking your pain and anger and directing it at those nearest you, well, frankly, who wants to be close to that? If most everything that comes out of your mouth is sharp, negative, judgmental, crude, abusive, or complaint-riddled, you become almost impossible to be emotionally active with.

Stop and listen to yourself during the course of the day. What do you hear? If you had to visualize your mood, are you more like: (A) A pleasant house with a well-kept lawn and a sunny welcome mat out front; or (B) A poorly maintained shack with junk scattered across your overgrown lawn and a Beware Of The Dog sign posted? Just think about it. Then do what you can to be more like choice A and less like choice B.

"Visualize your mood: are you a pleasant, welcoming house or a poorly maintained shack with a Beware Of The Dog sign posted?"

It's said that we need a core group—an inner circle—of about five very close friends. These are people we should try to talk to once a week. Our outer circle should consist of 50–100 acquaintances that we should try to talk to about once a year. Some of these are folks you see on and off, at your place of worship, favorite restaurant or bar, an old buddy from work, a girl who does your hair, a neighbor, or old schoolmate. The great news is it's easier now than ever to keep in touch. There's e-mail. There are social networking sites like Facebook. And now with Internet applications like Skype (a very cool, free, face-to-face, voice and video conversation program that we will discuss later), you can connect like never before.

Bottom line, being emotionally active is work, but don't be lazy in this regard. Like every other form of activity, take it slow. Don't keep it all bottled up. You'll find it's great to open up and share. Healthy, too.

✚ SEXUALLY ACTIVE

What?!!

It has come to my attention that some of you are not only dating again, but you're active under the sheets. I have one word for you: congratulations! Sexuality and physical intimacy are an important part of a healthy, vibrant life. There is no age limit for sex—especially now that many of you are taking advantage of new medications.

What does limit sexual activity, reports show, is how you feel physically. As overall health declines, so too does the prevalence of sexual activity. Said another way, an unhealthy side effect of poor health is a crummy sex life.

If you're returning to sexual activity, after perhaps a prolonged absence from intimacy, or because of the death of a long-term partner, lo and behold, the sparks, as well as the birds and the bees, do still fly. Be sure that the doctor in the mirror tells the Romeo or Juliet in the mirror to practice safe sex.

DR. YOU MEDICAL NOTE:

Sexually transmitted disease (STD) among older adults is rising at an alarming rate. Practice safe sex.

Of course, I don't mean protection from pregnancy. The concern is sexually transmitted disease (STD). As one senior said after becoming infected with HIV, "You never know the sexual history of anyone other than yourself." What she is telling you is to be safe. Unfortunately, there are people who have unprotected sex even though (knowingly or unknowingly) they have STDs. So be intimate, but be careful.

In fact, STDs among older adults are rising at an alarming rate. For example, incidence of syphilis increased a whopping 70% between 2005 and 2009 for those ages 55 to 64. Meanwhile, the incidence of chlamydia for that age group has risen 54%.[6]

Older adults are also the fastest-growing segment of the population living with HIV/AIDS. Be sure to use a condom. If you didn't already know this, there are both male and female condoms available at most drug stores. It's said the two most nervous people in a drug store are the teen buying condoms, and the senior making the same purchase. Yikes. Yes, it's a bit nerve-racking, but very necessary. If it's been some years since you used a condom, you should practice proper condom placement. Many informative, tastefully presented sources for help can be found online. That way when the lights are low, you're not learning as you go.

✚ PURPOSE IN LIFE

"I want to stay out of the nursing home."

"I want to stay independent."

"I don't want to be a burden."

As I travel across the country and meet people, these are declarations I hear all the time. Well, I don't mean to sound harsh, but I must ask: really? Do you really mean it? If your lifestyle includes bad habits, a poor diet, and very little physical and mental activity, you are on a crash course with health outcomes in direct opposition to your hopes and dreams.

My friends, being healthy takes work, discipline, and sacrifice. Those are qualities you possess and you have exhibited. It's time Dr. You took charge of what you can control and redirected your route.

Start by identifying one bad habit a month, and working to correct it. If you want freedom and independence in your later years, you have to fight for it now. Being healthy is patriotic. Quit smoking. Drink only in moderation. Improve your diet. Start small, with a new exercise routine customized from the ideas that we've just gone through.

The difference between someone who succeeds and someone who doesn't is often very simple: the successful person does what the unsuccessful person doesn't. Typically this is challenging because the easy way is rarely the best way. In fact, in hindsight, the easy way is often bland, soggy, and unrewarding. Yes, it's natural to be resistant and somewhat fearful of change. But you've handled change before and you can do it again.

"If your lifestyle includes bad habits, a poor diet, and very little physical and mental activity, you are on a crash course with health outcomes in direct opposition to your hopes and dreams."

The last third of your life can be your second childhood. Really. It can be a transformative time when you explore and draw new personal boundaries. Apprehension and fear are set aside so new interests and experiences can replace them. You have time again. Play. Exercise. Eat well. Live. Communicate. Stay in the game. Don't let life's pokes, prods, and challenges hold you back. Yes, you're going to be a bit creaky and slower and than you were in your first childhood. So what? Go for it. Find new purpose and joy in life.

Fill your calendar with activities. Feel the surge of confidence, the tingle of self-satisfaction, and the rush of pride that comes with being active. Discover this simple truth: when you get doing, you do yourself proud.

DOCTOR'S ORDERS
BE ACTIVE

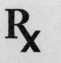

- Set goals for being active. It gives you greater purpose in life.

- Be active in three ways: physically, mentally, and socially.

- Don't let the "too" excuses keep you from being active: too much pain, too late for me, too busy, too expensive, too complicated, too hot, too cold.

- To customize your exercise routine, remember Six Butterflies Sipping Cocoa (SBSC): Stretch, balance, strength, and cardio.

- Try the medicine that doctors prescribe most: exercise!

- Get involved in group exercise; it's especially motivating.

- Exercise your brain by remaining mentally active.

- Leverage your "gray power." Collectively, the 55-plus population is a financial and political powerhouse.

Consult with your primary care physician before beginning a new exercise routine.

Dr. You

SECTION 2
MEDICAL DECISIONS

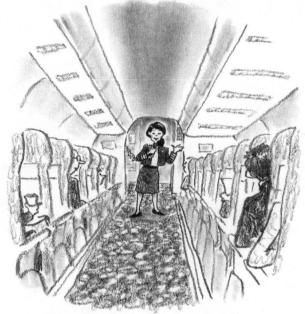

*"Is there a doctor on board?
No emergency, but mine's retiring."*

A few critical themes emerged from our first section. We talked about how Dr. You needs to get smart about diseases and their causes. You learned that you can control—and prevent—many chronic illnesses. And I hope it's now crystal clear that your lifestyle decisions are often the largest contributors to your illnesses and diseases. With most health circumstances you may face, you're not an innocent victim, nor should you be a helpless bystander. A big part of the remedy is in you becoming an engaged, enabled Dr. You.

"The best medical decision you can make is learning to get the health care system working as a team around you."

With age comes wisdom—it is true. Unfortunately, with age also comes increasing health issues. This next section will delve into how you can make the best medical decisions to deal with your conditions. Dr. You will learn how to effectively, efficiently manage the medical system so you can age with the maximum possible vitality and joy.

Here's a simple, yet profound, question: what is health? Dr. You needs to learn this answer, and then live it.

Here's how I define health. Health is not the absence of pain or disease. Health is an abundant sense of physical, mental, and spiritual well-being.

Let's break that down. Yes, statistics confirm that there will be pain, sickness, and disease as you age. But it's how you confront those challenges—and work to prevent new ones—that

DR. YOU MEDICAL NOTE:

Health is not the absence of pain or disease.
Health is an abundant sense of physical, mental, and
spiritual well-being.

will make you as physically, mentally, and spiritually healthy as
can be.

The theme of "what is health?" and exploring how to remain
healthy or return to health will be a prevailing concept as we
go forward in the book. Trust me, the concept of health as an
abundant sense of physical, mental, and spiritual well-being
should resonate deeper and deeper as we go forward.

In the chapters ahead, you will see how doctors, prescription medicine, hospitalization, and medical insurance will play a
larger role in life. How does Dr. You coordinate and orchestrate
these crucial parts of the medical system for optimal health?

I have a question for you, dear Reader. Would you say the
medical system is changing or remaining mostly the same? If
you answered "changing," you couldn't be more right. We'll talk
about how it's changing, why it's changing, and the best way to
leverage these major changes to better serve your health needs.

Making the best medical decisions may sound like a soli-
tary process: you go off to a mountaintop, think hard, wait for
an epiphany, and come back with a plan of action. Certainly
individual responsibilities are a part of sound medical decisions,

but in today's changing medical landscape, the operative word is *team*.

The next chapters will teach Dr. You how to organize your health team. You will learn how to get your primary physician, your surgeons, your specialists, your hospital, your pharmacist, your nurses, care managers, and other health professionals— even your family—working together in the name of your best health. This is your health circle. This is your health team.

The day of a lone Marcus Welby-type doctor toiling in isolation is ending. Our modern health care system can and should be a highly communicative network of professionals and facilities with Dr. You at the very center. This is known as patient-centric care: a type of care that is focused on your medical needs <u>and</u> your uniquely personal values. When patient-centric care is fully optimized, it's the best care in the world.

Those who want to age with vitality can't be passive and let the chips fall where they may with regard to medical decisions. Grab hold of the reins. You have to be a leader in assembling and communicating with your team. And you have to monitor its performance.

Speaking of performance, do you have the right primary care doctor for you? There is surprising variation in the quality of care delivered today. How is your patient-physician relationship? Do you *have* a patient-physician relationship? Are you doing your part to help your doctors? Do you know your essential medical data like blood pressure, cholesterol levels, and such? If you don't, there's a handy worksheet coming up called "Know Your Health in Numbers" that Dr. You needs to fill out.

Statistics show that as we age, living with multiple chronic illnesses and diseases becomes more and more a fact of life. Are your various doctors on the same page?

Do they all know what medications you're taking? Do you know what hospital is better for you depending on the condition that might bring you there? Have you ever done any homework to validate if one specialist or hospital is better than the next, or if you are using the best one for you?

PATIENT-CENTRIC CARE

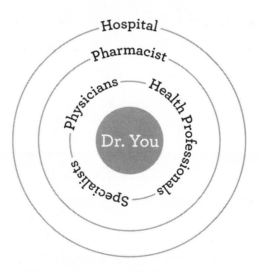

Organize your care around you

Dr. You is about to get very savvy when it comes to medical decisions. From clearly understanding everything from prescription drugs and your goals for taking them, to ensuring that your insurance plan is right for you, this section is filled with the simple tips and strategies you need.

Dr. You can't just sit back and cross your fingers and hope for the best. Patient-centric medicine means you're smack-dab in the middle of it. It all revolves around you.

Get educated. Get involved. Get what's best for you. That's what we'll be doing in this section. You need to initiate the conversation and collaborate in your health care decisions—after all, it is your quality of life we're talking about. Don't think of your medical care as doctors and nurses and caregivers scattered willy-nilly across a detached health care system. Think TEAM—with Dr. You in the center, actively making sure the right hand knows what the left hand is doing. That connectivity and synergy is how you get world-class quality care. And chances are, that's how the quality of your life will become worlds better, too.

CHAPTERS IN THIS SECTION:

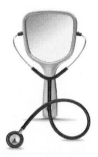

CHAPTER 5

DOCTOR VISITS

✚ "DING! DING! DING!" CHECK-UP TIME

Chances are, you've been seeing doctors for various health needs for many years. Through the span of these years, much has changed. Start with yourself; look at how you've changed. Look at how the car or transportation that takes you to your doctor's appointment has changed. Look at how the computers at the doctor's offices have changed. Despite change everywhere, have your expectations of your doctor changed? Or has the way you go about a doctor visit remained much the same?

Guess what, folks? It's time your doctor visits caught up with our changing times.

It's time to get the health care system working for Dr. You. This begins by placing yourself in the center of the process that we talked about called "patient-centric" care.

DR. YOU'S TOP FIVE REASONS FOR GOING TO A YEARLY CHECK-UP

1. Checking your blood pressure aids in the early detection of potential problems such as cardiovascular disease
2. Blood tests can help in the early detection of many potential illness and diseases before symptoms occur, particularly dangerously high cholesterol and diabetes
3. Other screenings, tests, and exams can detect diseases such as cancer early, when they are most treatable
4. Your physician can observe improvements or declines in health that occur too gradually for you to detect
5. It's your chance to communicate face-to-face with your doctor about any new or persistent health issues, and that could save your life!

First step: getting off the sidelines and into the game. Make an appointment for your annual check-up (and keep it!). I've heard all the excuses for not doing so: "I'm too busy." "My work schedule just won't allow it right now." "I feel great so I can skip a year." No, no, no. Tell yourself that a check-up can save your life, because you know what? It absolutely can. It's how doctors catch things early, when they're most treatable.

Have a look at Dr. You's top five reasons for going to a yearly check-up. And please, don't just keep this top five list to yourself. Encourage others to go to their yearly check-ups, too. Find a suitable way to tell them that this is more than a life-enhancing decision: it can be a life-saving decision. If someone were choking on a bite of food, would you just stand by? Of course not. Well, skipping regular check-ups can be just as dangerous.

It's often best not to attend your yearly check-up alone. If you can, bring a loved one or a friend (they can step out of the room at appropriate times). Why bother? Well, there can be a flood of information exchanged in a short period of time. Answers, treatments, and next steps can swirl together. By the time you get home, what was said can become as incomprehensible as a doctor's handwriting.

If you're alone, bring a pen and paper and take notes. Use the worksheets included in this chapter. More and more, the people I talk to are bringing a smart phone or e-tablet into the exam room to record a visit (with permission); don't be shy about asking. Good doctors all have one thing in common: they want and admire smart, informed patients.

Let me say one final thing about check-ups. We all know that seatbelts save lives—it's been proven over and over again. Most reasonable people would agree that they represent one of the more important safety improvements we've seen over

DR. YOU MEDICAL NOTE:

35% of those aged 65-plus skipped their flu shot. Yet, flu and pneumonia are the seventh-leading cause of death among older adults.

the course of our lives. Still, many of our generation often need a reminder to use seatbelts. You know, that annoying "Ding! Ding! Ding!" we hear when we forget to buckle up? Well, I want you to hear that same alarm if your annual check-up is overdue. You can hear it in your head. Or better yet, be the spouse, relative, or friend who serves as a nagging reminder to others that a check-up can save a life.

Mounting research suggests that married men live longer than single men, and it has been attributed in part to the fact that their wives nag them to go to the doctor. ("Ding! Ding! Ding!") And remember, Medicare and most insurance plans cover the cost of a yearly check-up, so there's no financial reason not to go.

Bottom line: Dr. You has to get involved. Don't be a mere passenger on the ship called health (remember the Titanic?). Climb into the wheelhouse and steer toward a better quality of life. Start by getting your check-up in the not-too-distant future. "Ding! Ding! Ding!"

+ IMMUNIZATIONS

Too many older Americans think vaccines are kids' stuff. That attitude can turn deadly. Yes, the flu (a virus) can be mild, but if you have other health conditions like diabetes or heart disease, it can quickly turn threatening. It's not uncommon for older adults who are weakened by fighting a flu virus to develop secondary infections such as pneumonia. We all know how dangerous pneumonia can be.

> **RECOMMENDED VACCINES TO DISCUSS WITH YOUR DOCTOR**
>
> - Influenza vaccine
> - Pneumococcal vaccine (pneumonia)
> - Tdap vaccine (tetanus, diphtheria, pertussis)
> - Zoster vaccine (shingles)

I just looked at some research reporting that between 40,000 and 50,000 adults die annually from vaccine-preventable diseases—including approximately 36,000 flu-related deaths annually.[1] Ninety-five percent of the flu-related deaths occur in adults 65-plus.[2] C'mon folks. This is dangerous stuff we're talking about!

The latest numbers show that approximately 60% of Americans ages 50-64 didn't get their influenza vaccine (flu shot). And about 35% of those age 65-plus also skipped their flu shot.[3] Yet, flu and pneumonia are the seventh-leading cause of death among older adults.[4] So in addition to getting your influenza vaccine, if you're 65-plus, I also recommend you get your pneumococcal vaccine, which protects against certain types of pneumonia.

There are a few things to know about your flu vaccine. There are two types: inactivated or "killed" vaccine, given by injection into the muscle; and live attenuated or "weakened" vaccine, sprayed into the nostrils.

The Centers for Disease Control and Prevention do not recommend nasal spray vaccinations to those 50 years of age and older. But if you're allergic to eggs, you should NOT get the shot, because eggs are used in making the vaccine. Talk to your doctor about alternative prevention.

The flu virus is very adaptive, changing constantly. That's why it's important to get your flu shot every year. Side effects from the shot are temporary, often lasting no more than a few days, including soreness, redness or swelling at the vaccination site, hoarseness, red, itchy eyes, cough, fever, and aches.

Remember, the shots are safe, and typically paid for by Medicare, so don't skip yours. By getting your vaccines you can protect yourself from a life-threatening illness. What's more, you'll be doing your community—including family, friends, children, and grandchildren—good by helping stop the spread of dangerous viruses.

One of the most common stories I hear is, "Dr. Reed, a few years ago I got my flu shot and within days I got the flu." I understand your concern. It's possible that you were already exposed to someone who had the flu virus by the time you got your shot, or that the flu-like illness you experienced was not the flu at all. The fact is, it's impossible to get the flu from the flu shot. Let me repeat: it's impossible to get the flu from the flu shot.

See the accompanying list of recommended vaccines to discuss with your doctor.

✚ KNOW YOUR HEALTH IN NUMBERS

We'll talk shortly about the quality of your physician, but first, how good are you at being a patient? Are you tuned into your health conditions and your needs?

"Why do people know the numbers of their favorite sports stars, but don't know their own blood pressure numbers?"

When talking to people, I'm always amazed to find out how few of them know their essential medical data. Why do people know the jersey numbers of their favorite sports stars, but don't know their own blood pressure numbers? How do you know the exact time and channel of your favorite TV dramas, but have no idea about your cholesterol numbers? You get the idea.

Maybe it's because no one told you it was important or made it easy for you to keep such a record. So now you have it right here in the book. Make a copy of the Know Your Health in Numbers worksheet included here. To complete it, look at your home health records or take it to your next physical and complete it there. Your physician will love working side-by-side with an eager new "white coat" called Dr. You.

Furthermore, for those of you like me who enjoy the latest in technology, you can now keep an electronic version of your personal health record in a secure, accessible location. This way

DOCTOR RESEARCH

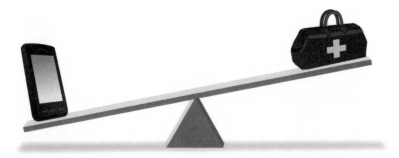

Most people spend more time researching their next electronic gadget than selecting their doctor

PATIENT HEALTH RECORD
KNOW YOUR HEALTH NUMBERS

Name:_____

Date:_____

Doctor & Clinic Information

Name:_____

Phone:_____

Pharmacy

Name:_____

Phone:_____

Pesonal Emergency Contact:

Name:_____

Phone:_____

1. My blood type is_____
2. Blood Pressure____ / ____
   a. BP Goal _____
3. Height _____
4. Weight _____
5. BMI (calculation) _____
6. Glucose/Sugar _____
7. Cholesterol ____ ____ ____
   HDL   LDL   Total
8. Medical History of Parents & Siblings

   _____
   _____
   _____
   _____

9. Names of All Medications; Over-the-Counter, Prescriptions & Supplements

   _____
   _____
   _____
   _____

10. Names of Medical Professionals

    _____
    _____
    _____
    _____

11. Date of last vaccination:
    a. Flu _____
    b. Pneumonia _____
    c. Tetanus _____
    d. Shingles _____

12. Date of last screening:
    a. Colon _____
    b. Mammogram _____
    c. Bones _____
    d. Eyes _____
    e. Vision _____
    f. Hearing _____

13. Date of last Dental Cleaning: _____

14. Allergies: _____

    _____
    _____
    _____

you can easily share it with the doctors, hospitals, emergency medical personnel, pharmacies, and other professionals on your health team. Find out more by going to mayoclinic.com and typing "electronic personal health record" into the search bar.

> **"The quarterback of your health team is your primary care physician."**

No doubt about it, the future of health records is going this way fast—and I mean racecar fast. When I attended the 2011 Indy 500, thousands of spectators had personal electronic health records made instantly and securely available to the medical personnel at the race. It was such a success that there are plans do it at the Super Bowl in 2012.

✚ BUILDING THE BEST HEALTH TEAM

So we've established that the health care landscape is rapidly changing (it's not your father's health care) and that we are embarking on a new era of medicine known as patient-centric care. As a result, your best chance at a longer, healthier life comes from being active in the process, not passive. You need to assemble your health team. And guess who is head coach? Yep, Dr. You.

If you're not communicating, or worse yet, if you're a no-show in your health, the team is breaking down before it ever had a chance to shine. C'mon, coach.

Taking this team analogy a step further, as coach, you have to select your players. The first selection, the key player that you rely on foremost, is the quarterback.

> **QUESTIONS TO ASK YOURSELF ABOUT YOUR PRIMARY CARE PHYSICIAN**
>
> 1. Does your doctor fit your needs and personality?
> 2. Have you ever communicated your expectations to your doctor?
> 3. How does your doctor rate in the science and art of care delivered?
> 4. Does your doctor listen to and respect your questions and wishes?

The quarterback of your health team is your primary care physician (also known as your family doctor or family practitioner). Along with your quarterback, there are other players on your health team. To name a few: specialists you may be seeing, physician's assistants, nurse practitioners, nurse care managers, your pharmacist, physical therapist, hospital doctors and personnel, and your family. That's a big team, which is great, but it requires careful coordination by both Dr. You and your primary care doctor.

You know if your team is clicking or not by asking yourself these questions:

Does the team care about me?

Do they understand my goals of care?

Do they listen to me?

Can I understand what they are saying to me?

Do they value my input?

Can we communicate and work together as a team?

But before we go any deeper about the whole team, let's talk about perhaps the most important question. Do you have the right quarterback?

✚ EVALUATING YOUR PRIMARY CARE PHYSICIAN

Your primary care doctor is your health quarterback. Think back. How did you choose him or her? Did you end up with your doctor by luck (or un-luck) of the draw? More importantly, are you happy with your current situation?

If you're thinking, C'mon, it doesn't really matter, you're mistaken. Could you imagine a coach of a winning team thinking his quarterback doesn't really matter? That's a sure way to a losing season. How many losing seasons of health can you afford?

As the Chief of Medical Affairs of UnitedHealth Group, I'm privileged to listen to the good people of this country talk about their health care. When it comes to choosing a doctor, do you know what I've learned? Most of you spend more time researching your next electronic gadget than you do researching your doctor. I know that oftentimes a friend or family member may have been influential in your decision, but you still have to do your own homework. You have to think of yourself as a consumer of medicine, just like you are a consumer of an electronic gadget. Except choosing the right doctor has significantly more impact on your life (despite all the "earth-shattering" bells and whistles promised on the gadget).

> **"All relationships are a two-way street.**
> **Don't just rate your doctor;**
> **rate Dr. You's performance as well."**

The fact is, all doctors are not created equal—the same goes for dentists, pharmacists, and other health professionals. You'd be surprised to learn how much variation there is in quality of the medicine practiced. I'm sure they all set out for excellence. Unfortunately, not all of them arrived there.

Before I continue, let me say that I have the utmost respect and admiration for doctors. I am honored and privileged to be a member of this worthy profession. Doctors commit their lives to selfless hours of training and continued education. They are dedicated to the ideals of physician professionalism and the care and well-being of others—swearing the Hippocratic Oath to practice medicine ethically. It is one of the few jobs in the world that we literally can't live without.

That said, as I learned in medical school, and throughout my career, some doctors are stronger in certain skill sets than others. One physician might excel in lab work. Another in diagnosis. And yet another may distinguish herself in a certain specialty. The point is, in the world of medicine where excellence is variable, how do you find the best doctor for you? Here are a few questions to ask yourself about your primary physician.

One: What are you looking for in a doctor? Who best fits your needs and your personality? You are a special individual, shaped by years of unique experiences and relationships. Typically, when your doctor has a similar value system, when there's common ground between you, it's easier for you to connect and communicate. (Those with multiple and complex health issues—and who are particularly frail—may want to consider a geriatrician as a part of their health care team.)

This could mean the "Top Doc" on the cover of the local magazine isn't right for you. Truth be told, many media ratings of Top Docs turn out to be little more than a popularity contest—with some doctors paying for their inclusion. Instead, your choice should come down to what role you want your doctor to play. Are you looking for a trusted confidant to whom you can tell all? Or a doctor who is more spiritually attuned? How about a doctor who plays it straight by the book—direct, and crisply professional? How about a doctor who takes more of a teacher/coach approach? Or do you need a doctor who is a strict enforcer? Knowing what characteristics best fit you will help in your assessment of the doctor you have, and will also give you a better idea of what type of doctor you're looking for. (What quarterback will make your health team successful?)

> **"If no one else has told you this, let me be the first: you deserve the best possible doctor."**

Two: Have you ever communicated your expectations to your doctor? How else are doctors to know what you need? They are awfully intuitive, but mind-reading is not a board-certified specialty. Tell them! Once a doctor knows what you're expecting, he or she can often work toward making the necessary adjustments. As long as both parties remain respectful, this moment of resetting expectations will by no means be confrontational, or even go beyond mildly uncomfortable. (Hint: tell your doctor you'd like to talk to them about your expectations. Say, "It might prick a little, but it won't hurt!")

Three: Because the quality of physician care is variable—and because each of you has such unique needs—I'd like you to use two criteria when deciding if you have the right doctor for you: evaluate the science and the art of medicine delivered.

First, consider the science. How does your doctor perform on what I'll call "hard measures" such as compliance with the best evidence-based clinical practices? This means the care being delivered is consistent with the best available scientific guidelines. Much of this data is just starting to be collected, formalized, and made available. To see a pilot program doing so, go to www.careaboutyourcare.org, a website and project sponsored by the Robert Wood Johnson Foundation. You'll find a U.S. map that lets you drill down into specifics. Other sources that measure important standards of care are the National Committee for Quality Assurance (NCQA). Go to www.ncqa.org, click on Programs, then click on Recognition. To find physician licensing information and disciplinary information, go to AIM Doc Finder at www.docboard.org.

Second, how does your doctor rate in the art of medicine? This evaluation involves "softer measures" of the patient's experience with care. For example, how well does your doctor listen and communicate with you? How easy is it to get access to the doctor and staff? Are your unique needs, values, and opinions respected and honored? Once again, the formalization and sourcing of this information is getting more robust by the day.

The key point I want you to remember is that a wise and prudent Dr. You has to factor the science and the art of medicine into your doctor evaluations, and discuss this in partnership with your health team. And be ready to integrate more of these performance measures into your decision-making in the months and years to come.

DOCTOR VISIT PREPARATION WORKSHEET

- Write down your health goals and fears, then discuss
- Tell your doctor everything: don't be afraid of disapproval or being judged
- Don't be afraid to respectfully question your doctor
  Good doctors want engaged patients
- Bring a loved one or friend if possible
- Bring in all your medications and supplements
- Bring your "Know Your Health in Numbers" chart
- Discuss any recent health developments

✚ DOCTORS CAN LEAVE A PERSON TONGUE-TIED

Doctors can be intimidating without being aware of it. In fact, when a doctor begins your check-up and you're told to open your mouth and say "ahhh," you know what the doctor often finds? You're tongue-tied. "Ahhh" might be your first and last spoken word!

What you both need to work on is undoing that knot in your tongue so you can communicate openly, honestly, and productively. Ask questions. If a doctor prescribes a test, a

> **DR. YOU MEDICAL NOTE:**
>
> It's best not to attend your yearly check-up alone. Bring a loved one or a friend to record important results, advice, and next steps.

screening, or a procedure, ask why. If the answer doesn't sound right, or is confusing, politely and respectfully let your doctor know. A doctor won't be offended by your active participation in your health. If your doctor refuses to answer your question, or can't give you evidence-based reasoning for a decision, then you need to find a new doctor. Period.

"Get your doctor to listen to more than your heart and lungs. Express your goals and fears."

Equally imperative is that you get your doctor to listen to more than your heart and lungs. Express your goals and fears. For example, if you're worried that your chronic leg pain is becoming more and more immobilizing, but your goal is to be active enough to go whitewater rafting with your visiting grandchildren, let your doctor know. This way you can get a medical opinion on the viability of your goal, and begin working on a plan to make it a reality. This is a relationship, not a passive procedure. You should go away from every doctor visit feeling empowered and excited about your health goals.

✚ A HEALTHIER RELATIONSHIP

It takes two to tango. As we go about evaluating the capabilities of your primary physician, I'd suggest you keep in mind that all relationships are a two-way street. Don't just rate your doctor's performance, also rate Dr. You. Are you completely honest and open? Are you listening? Are you following prescribed treatment? Are you tuned into your health conditions and your needs? Are you living up to your half of the bargain during your doctor visits?

Take a moment to assess the relationship you have with your primary doctor. Give it a letter grade, just like in school, from A to F: A is excellent, B is very good, C is adequate, D is poor, and F is failing. Stop and really think about it for a moment… come up with the letter grade that your patient-physician relationship has earned. Okay, pencils down.

If you earned an A or B, congratulations. You have a great thing going. Keep it up. If you gave your relationship a C, D, or F, it's time for a change in one form or another. Let me explain why the change doesn't always involve switching primary physicians.

If you gave the relationship a C, the first change to make is how you communicate with your doctor. Explain your needs and expectations more clearly, with the hope of lifting that grade to a B or better. I'd like you to assume something called "positive intent" of your physician. That is, your doctor wants to do what's beneficial and in your health's best interest, but he or she may need a little help from you. Oftentimes all it takes is an open, honest conversation.

If your relationship scored a D or an F, it's time to begin looking for a new primary care doctor. It may be no one's fault in particular, but you and your doctor are simply not a good match. It's not the end of the world, but it should be the end of the relationship.

If no one else has told you this, let me be the first: you have the right to the best possible doctor. It's your body and your life. You are a one-of-a-kind miracle. Be sure you get the special attention and respect you're entitled to. If it's time for a change, it's time for a change. Let's talk more about how to go about it, and why you shouldn't be afraid to do so.

✚ "I THINK I NEED TO CHANGE DOCTORS"

The notion of changing doctors is a scary thought. While I realize that change is rarely easy, it is, at times, necessary. Your health is at stake—possibly, at some point, even your life.

DR. YOU MEDICAL NOTE:

Give your patient-doctor relationship a letter grade from A (excellent) to F (failing).

If your attempts at clearer, more productive communication and your polite requests for closer attention to your medical needs have resulted in no measurable change, start your search for a new doctor. I believe that this country is blessed with more great doctors than any other in country the world.

Sometimes making a change isn't your choice. Unfortunately, favorite doctors do retire. Doctors also occasionally move away, making it no longer practical to remain under their care.

So how do you find the right doctor for you? Check with your health insurer. You can find out what doctors are in your network, and some insurers also provide physician quality ratings. You can also ask your nurses. If you politely whisper to them during an appointment that you're thinking of changing doctors, they could very likely make a good suggestion or two. Word-of-mouth referrals from family, friends, or trusted acquaintances can be productive, too.

Dear Reader, I'd be remiss if I didn't mention one final observation about changing doctors. If you notice that you're constantly changing, that you're never satisfied, and that this behavior pattern of dissatisfaction exists not only with doctors, but in many other facets of life, it may be wise to stop for a moment and have a look in the mirror. Maybe the doctor who needs to change is Dr. You.

✚ YOU DESERVE A GREAT DOC

As you age, you tend to need more health care, and the care required often becomes increasingly complex. As a result, your primary doctor—your health care quarterback—becomes more and more critical.

Don't suffer through a poor relationship with your doctor. If attempts to improve this partnership are going nowhere, make a change. You need to max your doc.

"You need to max your doc!"

In your lifetime, chances are your primary physician will be called on to coordinate multi-source care. Say, for example, you have a complicated case of diabetes. That could mean adding an endocrinologist to your team. Say the endocrinologist wants you to eat a special diet and get more exercise to manage your diabetes. Now you might add a nutritionist and physical therapist to your team. The orchestration of that care starts with Dr. You and your primary physician. An open, honest, friendly dialogue between everyone involved is crucial—beginning with you and your primary physician. If you're constantly walking on eggshells, or afraid to ask questions or make requests, your health will suffer.

Furthermore, statistics show that more and more of us are working past retirement age. As a result, work-related injuries are on the rise among those in their 60s and beyond. Add to that our higher expectations for longer lives than those of previous generations, and you can see why a primary physician is important like never before.

What I'm saying is don't just settle. You deserve greatness. And greatness is out there ready to serve you.

✚ OTHER DOCTOR VISITS

One of the oldest jokes in the book is, *Have you seen your optometrist lately? If you haven't, you'll be seeing even less of him in the future.* (Get it?)

A few other doctors I'd like to remind you to set appointments with are your optometrist (or ophthalmologist), your audiologist, and your dentist.

If you're 65-plus, have your eyes checked every year. An eye exam can lead to important corrections to your prescription, which helps your everyday life—particularly when driving. More importantly, it can be the source of early detection of cataracts, glaucoma, macular degeneration, and other eye diseases that can lead to blindness. You can go to www.eyecareamerica.org to see if you qualify for a free exam.

By age 60, be sure to have your hearing tested, too. Depending on your hearing health or your work environment, your doctor may recommend that you see an audiologist sooner than this.

If you're putting off having your hearing tested, I'd like you to consider a few things. Poor hearing is frustrating for those on both sides of the conversation. Plus it's unsafe. To know what direction sounds are coming from, and to be able to accurately identify them, is essential to safety—especially while driving or when walking in congested areas.

"My father was a dentist. He saw first-hand the critical role a healthy smile played in the quality of a person's life."

Oftentimes, poor hearing is nothing more than wax buildup, which is easily corrected by having your ears flushed at your yearly check-up. There are also a number of eardrops available for in-home use. If it is more than wax buildup, there are many virtually invisible hearing products that can have you hearing sounds that you've been missing for years. The quality of your relationships (and your confidence) can benefit greatly from better hearing.

Finally, let's not forget about 32 (give or take a few) of the best friends or worst enemies a person can have: your teeth. Make an appointment to see the dentist. Poor oral health can lead to painful decay and infections, as well as diminished self-esteem and difficulty in social situations. Doctors have even found links between poor oral health and heart disease.

My father was a dentist. He saw first-hand the critical role a healthy smile played in the quality of a person's life. From enabling you to eat healthy, nutritious food that requires rigorous chewing to presenting an outward sign of good hygiene and sparkling health, your smile plays a center-stage role in life. Be sure to get to the dentist once or twice a year, brush at least twice daily, and floss at least once a day. It's a small investment in one of your most noticeable attributes. Plus, our world could use a few more smiling faces.

DOCTOR'S ORDERS
DOCTOR VISITS

R_X

- "Ding! Ding! Ding!" Get your yearly check-up. Early detection of a disease can save your life.

- Get your immunizations, have your hearing and eyesight checked, and see your dentist at least once a year.

- Bring a loved one or friend to doctor appointments to write things down.

- In this era of "patient-centric health care," you need to be the coach of your whole health team.

- Your primary care physician (PCP) is the quarterback of your heath care team. Keep an honest line of communication open.

- Do your homework when choosing your doctor. Most people spend more time researching their next electronic gadget than selecting a doctor.

- It's vital that you "Know Your Health in Numbers" and monitor this essential health data with your doctor.

- Evaluate your doctor on the science and art of care delivered.

- Good doctors welcome questions and are not offended when you get a second opinion of a diagnosis.

Dr. You

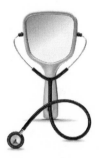

CHAPTER 6

PRESCRIPTION DRUGS AND MEDICATIONS

✚ THE MANY TYPES AND FORMS OF MEDICATION

We live in amazing times. Some of the world's foremost scientists and researchers are working around the clock, discovering and developing miraculous medications to enhance and save lives. As a result, the range of pharmaceuticals available today is unprecedented.

Let's begin by looking at broad categories of drugs. First, there are drugs commonly known as prescription drugs that can only be obtained with a written prescription from your doctor—these come labeled as brand-name drugs and generic drugs.

DR. YOU MEDICAL NOTE:

Think of your medications as a whole—as a totality—and be wary of potentially dangerous interactions that each drug can cause when taken with another. No exceptions.

Then there are over-the-counter (OTC) medications, which the Food and Drug Administration has deemed safe and appropriate for use without a prescription. These also come in brand names and generics.

And the last group of medications we'll talk about are dietary supplements, including vitamins, minerals, herbs, and others.

Regardless of the category of medications that you're taking, you need to be careful. Every drug is powerful and potentially dangerous on its own, and even more so when mixed with other medicines. What this means is Dr. You has to think of your medications as a whole—as a totality—and be wary of potentially dangerous interactions that each drug can cause when taken with another. No exceptions.

✚ KNOW YOUR STUFF

Dr. You needs to become a medication know-it-all. To begin, Google each medication that you take and learn about it. What's the active ingredient? Is it a brand-name drug, or are

DR. YOU MEDICAL NOTE:

From 1999 to 2009, the number of prescriptions filled in America increased by almost 40%.

you taking the generic version? What side effects should you be on the lookout for?

Let me take a minute to explain the difference between brand-name and generic drugs. Generally speaking, when a new medication is developed, the drug company makes significant investments of time and money—as well as adhering to a rigorous regulatory approval process. As a result, when the new drug compound is approved, the manufacturer gets the right to put their brand name on it and have an exclusive right to sell it for a protected period of time—typically seven years. After that time, the compound becomes available as a generic, which means other manufactures can make the same formulation. As a result, typically the drug becomes more affordable.

The key thing for you to know is that in almost every instance, the generic formulation of the compound is the same as the brand-name formulation. However, from time to time your physician may decide that for some special reason you should take the specific brand formulation of the drug. Otherwise, the generic is just as good. And usually less expensive.

The next thing to get smart on is the possibility of dangerous interactions between your drugs. Of course, talk to your physician and pharmacist about this issue. You can also go to www.drugdigest.org. It's a trusted, simple website where you can search a menu of medications to find out how drugs interact with each other and with foods and alcohol. Talk to your doctor about any worrisome results you see.

QUESTIONS TO ASK WHEN YOUR DOCTOR PRESCRIBES A MEDICINE

- What is the name of my medication, and is there a generic version?
- What condition(s) does my medication treat?
- How and when should I take my medication?
- For how long should I take my medication, and if I feel better, do I need to finish the entire amount of medication as prescribed?
- What are the risks associated with the medication and do the benefits outweigh those risks? What are the alternatives? (For example: Does my medication contain anything that can cause an allergic reaction? Should I expect any side effects from my medication?)
- Are there any foods, drinks, or activities I need to avoid while taking this medication?
- Is it safe for me to take this medication with other medications or dietary supplements?
- How soon will this medicine start working?
- What should I do if I miss a dose of my medication?
- Will any tests be necessary while I am taking this medication?

All medications have the potential to interact dangerously with each other and even with your other medical conditions. Don't think, for example, that an OTC drug can't interact with another OTC drug—it can! Often in very complex ways. We'll talk shortly about the necessity of Dr. You getting all your medications together and going over them with your physician and pharmacist. And that includes multivitamins and dietary supplements (calcium or glucosamine supplements, for example) and all natural herbs like St. John's Wort. Discuss all of this with your doctor and pharmacist. Just because it's a supplement or labeled "all natural" doesn't mean it won't interact negatively with your meds. As you may know from many news stories, supplements are not as well regulated as prescription and OTC medications are, so be extra careful.

✚ HAVE GOALS FOR YOUR MEDICATIONS

There can be no question: breakthrough medicines have improved the quality of many of our lives. Prescription medicines, for example, along with other medical advances, have helped lower death rates for heart disease, stroke, cancer, HIV/AIDS, and other diseases.

That said, dear Reader, you have to be careful about how you use them. With every prescription drug you take, you need to have simple goals for that medication.

Your first goal, as we just talked about, is to understand your medicine. Be it brand, generic, OTC, supplements—whatever—know your stuff. Please remember, you don't have to do this all alone. For example, when you're seeing your doctor, bring a loved one or friend if possible. Oftentimes, medications are prescribed after a difficult medical event like surgery. It's hard to comprehend everything being said. Write medication instructions down. A friend or loved one in the room can assist you, and help you grasp and remember all the details of your treatment. Ask questions. If the answers are unclear, politely ask for clarification.

Your second goal is to get your prescription filled. Sound easy? One would think so, but according to the National Consumers League, 25 to 33% of prescriptions never get filled. And even when they are filled, only about 50% of patients take their medicine as prescribed. How is your medicine supposed to help you if you don't take it properly?

This leads us to your third goal, which is to take the medicine as directed: the dosage, the frequency, and the length of time. More about that in a moment.

Your fourth and final goal is to understand how your medication fits into your entire treatment plan, including, for example, physical therapy, diet, and exercise.

For a rational and prudent Dr. You, the reason why you're taking a medication should never be, "because my doctor told me to." You need to have a clear-cut understanding and simple goals for each medication. What I'm getting at, and it's probably not going to win me any popularity contests, is that too many people today wash down a pill with complacency, or worse yet, ignorance. That needs to end.

> **DR. YOU MEDICAL NOTE:**
>
> To find out if your drugs could have possible dangerous interactions, go to www.drugdigest.org. Also talk to your doctor and pharmacist.

There are many smart questions to ask. To get started, use those suggested on the chart provided called Questions to Ask When Your Doctor Prescribes a Medicine. It really helps you understand your medicine and keep to your goals. Think of it this way: don't just take a pill, take control.

"Adhere to regimens. How is your medicine supposed to help you if you don't take it properly?"

✚ ADHERE TO REGIMENS

Start by reading the label!

Sorry to blurt at you, but I talk to people all the time who don't read the medication instructions on the label. It makes me crazy. Please, take your meds as directed.

Dr. You needs to know your drug regimen—and stick to it. If your prescription instructs that you take two pills, that means take two. I can't tell you the number of people who give me a little wink and say, "Psst, Dr. Reed. I cut my prescription in half to save money." That's a darn fast way to render your medication ineffective. (And it's a poor use of your hard-earned money!) Did you know that a drug's active ingredient isn't always dispersed evenly in the pill? The only time that it's okay for you cut a pill in half is when it's been scored by the manufacturer (scoring is the indented line across the pill). Always consult your doctor or pharmacist before doing so.

"Think of it this way: don't just take a pill, take control."

By the same token, adhering to regimens means you cannot take an extra dose to offset an unusual amount of pain on a particular day, unless approved by your doctor. And also be sure to finish the full course of any prescribed antibiotics, even after you feel better. Otherwise you run the risk of helping create drug-resistant infections for yourself, your community, your children, and your grandchildren. This is how we got the drug-resistant bugs you hear so much about in the media today. Please, let's not create more of them. Remember: finish off the antibiotic, finish off the bacteria.

MEDICATION TIPS

- No medicine is completely safe. It's approved by the FDA when the FDA judges that the benefits of the medicine outweigh the known risks for the labeled use

- Use a pill box marked with the days of the week because it's easy to confuse pill bottles—especially when in a rush

- Stick a reminder note on your bathroom mirror

- Keep your medicine in a place where you will see it daily

- Plan ahead for refills. For example, mark a calendar with a "Refill on" date

- Pick up refills the week before your medicine runs out

- Make sure you have enough refills to last until your next doctor visit

- Check with your pharmacy to see if it offers an automatic refill service

- If your medicine is ordered by mail, order refills at least two weeks in advance

- Regarding the cost of medicines: most health plans offer mail order services and programs designed to reduce costs for members. Also ask your plan about any available coupon programs to lower costs

- Medication can leave you constipated. Drink plenty of water and ask your doctor or pharmacist about suggested stool softeners or laxatives

- When comparing medication treatments for common diseases, go to ahrq.gov and click on the Consumer & Patients section for helpful information

- If you feel like you're taking too many medications, two actions are proven effective in reducing the number: becoming more knowledgeable about your meds, and lifestyle changes such as increased activity or changes in diet

Why don't people take prescriptions as directed? What are the barriers? I ask people this all the time. Some just shrug their shoulders, which tells me they're not respecting the consequences of taking medication. Maybe it's because some pills are small and taken frequently—it becomes so routine that they don't think about it.

Some folks are forgetful. Others are too busy. Here's where Dr. You has to take action. Use a dated organizer pillbox. Set watch alarms. Leave notes on the mirror in the bathroom. There are a number of new devices—from vibrating pocket alarms to programmable automatic medication dispensers—to help you to stay on regimen.

And remember, it's *your* regimen, not someone else's. Everyone's body reacts uniquely to medication. Dr. You may know your own medicines, but you're not qualified to start dispensing treatment to others. Never take anyone else's prescription, or give them yours.

Let's say your spouse wrenched her back and was given a prescription that worked great for her pain. Now, let's say you hurt your knee—do not take her pain medication. It might not be the right drug or dose for you. And you might have medical conditions that contradict the use of this medication, or you could be taking other meds that might cause a dangerous interaction. You don't know. And this is not the time to gamble.

DR. YOU MEDICAL NOTE:

An unfilled prescription or a medication not taken can dangerously unbalance your treatment and confuse your medical team.

Here's another situation to watch out for: you begin a regimen of a particular medication, but you can't tolerate it. For example, if the medicine makes you feel sick, dizzy, or sleepy, notify your doctor right away. Or if you're prescribed a medication and for some reason—let's say cost—you don't intend to take it. Again, you must have an honest conversation with your doctor as soon as possible. An unfilled prescription or a medication not taken can dangerously unbalance your treatment and confuse your medical team. You'll read more on the importance of a fully informed, coordinated health team shortly

✚ A PILL FOR EVERY ILL?

I want to warn you to be careful with medications and equally careful about your attitude toward them. Don't think of medications as inherently good or bad. They have to be assessed, person by person, condition by condition. At this moment in medicine, although, I'm not sure that enough doctors or patients are pausing to consider all the treatments available to fight disease. And too often, they don't know what medications other doctors have prescribed. As a result, the prescriptions are piling on.

I've spoken with some experts on this subject and the numbers they offer are not encouraging. As we age and experience more chronic diseases, we often require more chronic medication. Approximately 65% of Americans 60-plus require three or more drugs per day, and almost 40% require five or more drugs per day.[1] Not only is that percentage on the rise, but the number of drugs being used is expanding, too. For example, from 1999 to 2009, the number of prescriptions increased almost 40%.[2]

Why is the use of prescription, over-the-counter, and herbal medications climbing?

As I said, chronic illnesses are rising. But frankly, many of us are unwilling to tolerate discomfort, so we try to "solve it" with medication. As a culture we've slipped into a "pill for every ill" mentality.

Part of this mentality is due to a heightened awareness of drugs. Drug companies are powerful marketers. You can't have a symptom these days without turning around and bumping into a drug promoted to treat it. Our culture needs to rethink medication. Turn off the TV commercials and flip past the magazine advertisements. Instead of listening to paid actors selling you on what medication you need, listen to Dr. You. Then have a thoughtful conversation with your doctor.

Set goals for your medication. Share those goals with family and loved ones. Find the minimum medications you need for maximum health—no more, no less. And get on with a happy, productive life.

✚ SIDE EFFECTS

There's a term in the world of prescription drugs known as a "medication misadventure." It refers to an adverse drug effect, such as an unintended or dangerous reaction to a medicine.

PILL FOR EVERY ILL?

40%

65%

Approximately 65% of Americans 60-plus require three or more drugs per day; almost 40% require five or more drugs per day

We certainly don't want a medication that causes more harm than good. That may sound overly obvious, yet the frequency of medication side effects is alarming. Did you know that almost 10% of hospital admissions are due to drug side effects and medicine misadventures?[3] So here's a two-part approach that I want you to use when addressing the subject of side effects with your doctor.

First, ask if there are any side effects that should cause you to stop taking the medication <u>immediately</u>. For example, if you were taking a cholesterol-lowering medication, the side effects could include things like an allergic reaction, leg cramps, or flu-like muscle aches.

Second, discuss other side effects that you should be aware of, and how to respond. For example, your doctor may tell you that your prescribed antibiotic may cause an upset stomach, but try to keep taking the drug and lessen the side effect with toast or other light food. Then communicate any changes.

My advice: before taking a medication, first open your mouth and ask questions. And keep opening your mouth to ask follow-up questions until satisfied. Remember our theme for this chapter: don't just take a pill, take control.

Speaking of side effects, there is a medication complication called the "prescribing cascade" that you should watch out for. In short, what happens is this: you're prescribed a medicine, which causes a side effect, which is then treated with another medicine, which causes a new side effect, which is treated with yet another medicine—and on and on it goes. This cascading can continue to snowball with dangerous results. So it's vital that you know what side effects to look out for, and to communicate any new symptoms as a result of a medication regimen.

And remember those dangerous interactions that we've been talking about? Here's a common example: the popular over-the-counter heartburn pill Prilosec® reduces the effectiveness of Plavix®, an anti-clotting medicine taken by over 80 million people. This unintended consequence can raise the risk of heart attack and strokes in people taking Plavix. Lesson for Dr. You: by taking what I once heard a woman call an "innocent over-the-counter medicine," you can jeopardize your

BROWN BAG IT!

LOIS'S
MEDS

Once a year gather all your medications—
of any kind—and bring them in to your primary
doctor for review

heart medicine's effectiveness, and even your life. This is why your health team needs to know all the medications that you're taking. All as in all.

Here are two other examples of harmful interactions: OTC medications like aspirin or ibuprofen can dangerously increase the chances of bleeding in people taking anti-clotting medications like Coumadin®. And using OTC nasal decongestants can cause elevated blood pressure.

My point is, there is no such thing as an innocent over-the-counter medicine. Just because a prescription wasn't required for the medicine doesn't mean it's inconsequential, especially to the effects of other drugs. What we see—sometimes after a frightening (and expensive) trip to the ER—are patients who didn't realize that OTC medications could increase or decrease the effectiveness of other drugs, or increase certain side effects. Many folks have to learn this the hard way. Do friends and family a favor instead, and pass this information on.

Two final notes of caution. Some drugs (such as warfarin, digoxin, and seizure medication) require frequent monitoring of blood levels. This may involve additional lab work for you, but stick to it. Remember the unplanned visits to the ER we talked about earlier? You don't want to join that group. Also see the included list of medications that older adults should be cautious of or avoid entirely. If you find one of your medications on the list, talk to your doctor and pharmacist and tell them that you're concerned.

✚ MAKING A LIST AND CHECKING IT TWICE

A few months ago I gave a talk. Afterward I was chatting with a spry older gentleman. He had a gleam in his eye when he told me that he was busier than most seniors—then he paused a beat for comedic timing—most *high school* seniors! We had a good laugh. But it reminded me how jam-packed days can get.

WAYS TO SAVE MONEY ON PRESCRIPTION MEDICATIONS

1. Ask your doctor or pharmacist. Your doctor may know of local or national programs to help
2. State and local government programs may offer help. Check out your state's website or contact your representative. See also: www.medicare.gov/Publications/Pubs/pdf/10126.pdf, and www.socialsecurity.gov, click on Medicare, then click on Get extra help with Medicare drug plan costs
3. Shop for the lowest price. Prices can vary widely. Just be cautious about buying from multiple sources—one source is best for monitoring drugs for potentially dangerous interactions
4. Consider using U.S. mail-order services. Patients usually can order up to a 3-month supply of prescription medicine for a lower cost than individual prescription refills
5. Pharmaceutical assistance programs. Most pharmaceutical companies now have programs to help lower-income patients or those with no insurance coverage. Contact the Partnership for Prescription Assistance by phone (1-888-4PPA-NOW) or on the Web at www.pparx.org

---

DR. YOU MEDICAL NOTE:

Pharmacists are drug experts. They went to school and studied drugs longer than most physicians.

You have a busy life with a lot of daily details to manage—not the least of which is your prescriptions. Medications and dosages can change. It can get confusing—in a hurry. Write down all your medications including: prescriptions, OTC, dietary supplements like multivitamins, calcium, herbals, fish oil, even medication like eye drops, topical creams, inhalers, and nebulizers. Use the My Medicine List chart provided here (or make a photocopy). Also copy your list on to a smaller piece of paper to be kept in your wallet or purse in case of an emergency. A list like that can come in handy, for example, if you're traveling and you end up at a different pharmacy. And as we talked about earlier, for you tech-savvy readers, this list of medications would be included on your electronic personal health record.

Here are a few tips for the next time you jump on an plane headed for some exciting destination: keep your medications with you and not in your checked luggage because you never know where your bags will end up, right? Bring more than enough medication for your trip. Review your dosage schedule before you leave and determine if you need to make any time zone changes. And double-check your wallet to be sure your list of medications is there and up to date.

In recent years, medical alert bracelets have become a more common way to record your medications and conditions. In case of an emergency, when you can't speak for yourself, these bracelets and necklaces are invaluable. And thanks to their attractive designs, they are pretty stylish, too.

Let me give you a life-saving scenario: a woman is taking the blood-thinner Coumadin® for a blood clot issue. She's in a car accident and loses consciousness. Her engraved med alert bracelet has a concise overview of her conditions and medications. The EMTs and first responders, who are trained to look for these bracelets, promptly alter their treatment protocol based on this new information, increasing the chances of a best outcome.

I have a friend who wears a sterling silver necklace identifying him as a diabetic who is insulin-dependent. It also communicates his drug allergies, along with a preferred hospital and emergency contact. This is information that you don't want medical professionals guessing about when they treat you under time-sensitive conditions.

✚ SINGLE SOURCE

You may be familiar with the phrase "the right hand needs know what the left hand is doing." What this means in the context of your meds is if multiple doctors are writing multiple prescriptions, all doctors involved need to be aware of all the medications that you're taking.

I heard from a nurse the other day whose patient was in the ER twice over the past two weekends. As it turns out, her patient—who had a heart condition—was unknowingly taking a double dose of beta blockers: both the brand name and the generic. One prescription was written by her cardiologist, the other by her primary physician, without any knowledge of the other. Folks, this is an extremely dangerous situation. You need to get all your doctors and your pharmacist on the same page by sharing an up-to-date copy of your master drug list. Your life can depend on it.

I also suggest that at least once a year you "brown bag it"—especially if you've had a recent hospitalization. Gather up all your medication bottles—of any kind—put them in a brown lunch sack, and bring all of them in to your primary doc. This helps everyone know exactly what you're taking.

Furthermore, try to get all prescriptions filled at a single pharmacy or pharmacy chain if possible. This way, there's a greater chance of detecting any potential problems ahead of time.

And last but certainly not least, don't overlook the important role that your pharmacist can play on your health team. Pharmacists are medication experts. They went to school and studied drugs longer than most physicians. Talk to them frequently and use them wisely regarding your medications and their most effective use.

OLDER ADULTS SHOULD BE CAUTIOUS OF OR AVOID THESE MEDICATIONS

- Non-steroidal anti-inflammatory drugs (NSAIDs). Examples: piroxicam (sold under the brand-name Feldene®) and indomethacin (Indocin®)
- Muscle relaxants. Examples: cyclobenzaprine (Flexeril®), methocarbamol (Robaxin®), carisoprodol (Soma®) and similar medications
- Anti-anxiety and anti-insomnia drugs. Examples: benzodiazepines, such as diazepam (Valium®), alprazolam (Xanax®) or chlordiazepoxide (Librium®, Limbitrol®, Librax®) as well as sleeping pills, such as zaleplon (Sonata®) and zolpidem (Ambien®)
- Anticholinergic drugs. Examples: medications including the antidepressants amitriptyline (Elavil®) and imipramine (Tofranil®), the anti-Parkinson's drug trihexyphenidyl (Artane®), the irritable bowel syndrome drug dicyclomine (Bentyl®), and the overactive bladder drug oxybutynin (Ditropan®)
- Heart medication. Example: digoxin (Lanoxin®) in doses greater than 0.125 mg
- Diabetes drugs. Example: glyburide (Diabeta®, Micronase®) and chlorpropamide (Diabinese®)
- Opioid pain relievers. Examples: meperidine (Demerol®) and pentazocine (Talwin®)
- Anti-psychotic drugs. Examples: Unless you are being treated for schizophrenia, bipolar disorder or some forms of depression, stay away from anti-psychotics such as haloperidol (Haldol®), risperidone (Risperdal®) and quetiapine (Seroquel®)
- Estrogen. Example: Estrogen pills and patches, which are typically prescribed for hot flashes and other menopause-related symptoms
- Over the counter (OTC) medications: Especially antihistamines chlorpheniramine (AllerChlor®, Chlor-Trimeton®) and diphenhydramine (which is used in sleep aids including Tylenol PM® as well as in cold and allergy brands such as Benadryl®). They can cause confusion, blurred vision, constipation, urination problems, and dry mouth in older adults

DOCTOR'S ORDERS
PRESCRIPTION DRUGS AND MEDICATIONS

- Get your prescriptions filled and take your medications as directed.

- Have goals for your medications, including knowing how they fit in with your entire treatment plan.

- Put all your medications, supplements, and herbal products in a bag and bring them to your next doctor visit.

- When a drug is prescribed, ask if alternative non-pharmaceutical treatments are available. (To name a few: exercise, diet adjustments, massage, and acupuncture.)

- Be sure if multiple doctors are writing multiple prescriptions, all doctors involved are aware of all the medications that you're taking.

- Know what drugs older adults should be cautious of or avoid. (See the chart in this chapter.)

- When traveling, keep your medications with you and not in your checked luggage.

- Pharmacists are medication experts. They are a great resource for questions about drugs and their most effective use.

Dr. You

MY MEDICINE LIST

Name:	D.O.B:	Allergic To: *(Describe reaction)*

Emergency Contact/Phone numbers:

Doctor(s):

Pharmacies, other sources:

Immunization Record *(Record the date/year of last dose taken)*

	Flu vaccine(s):	
Pneumonia vaccine:	Tetanus:	Hepatitis vaccine:	Other:

List all medicines you are currently taking. Include prescriptions (examples: pills, inhalers, creams, shots), over-the-counter medications (examples: aspirin, antacids, vitamins) and herbals (examples: ginseng, gingko). Include medications taken as needed (example: nitroglycerin, inhalers).

START DATE	NAME OF MEDICATION DOSE	DOSE	DIRECTIONS *(How do you take it? When? How Often?)*	DATE STOPPED	GOALS *(Reason for taking?)*

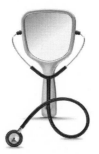

CHAPTER 7

HOSPITALIZATION

✛ A HEALING STATE OF MIND

When I ask people if they're prepared to go to the hospital they give me an anxious look and say, "What? Is something wrong?" I assure them that no, nothing is wrong... at the moment. But as the Boy Scouts have preached since 1910: Be Prepared.

"Prepare for the hospital?" you might say. "Why? Something bad happens. You go to the hospital. Where's the preparation in that?"

Exactly. Where's the preparation in that?

Let's back up a minute and look at this from a broader perspective. Dr. You has been preparing since page one of this book. You've learned to make adjustments in behavior, diet, and activity levels to prevent disease and promote health. And you know how to assemble your health team and get them on the same page with your medications and treatments.

"An expert on the subject told me that hospital patients will function at a fifth- to seventh-grade level during recovery."

Yet despite these best efforts to be as healthy and happy as can be, it's a very rare bird who is born in the hospital and never looks back. In fact, like it or not, as we age, most of us will spend multiple days in the hospital. Preparation is key. You want to end up in the right hospital to meet your needs, and make your stay there as short and productive as possible. The goal is to be in a healing state of mind, and preparation plays a big role in that.

One way to prepare is to decide what type of patient you will be, lying in the hospital bed. You can be a helpless patient or an enabled Dr. You. Yes, there will very likely be a window of time that you will need significant help. In fact, an expert on the subject told me that patients typically function at a fifth- to seventh-grade level during hospital recovery. But there is time before and after that window where you can ably do for yourself.

> **DR. YOU MEDICAL NOTE:**
>
> For best outcomes, approach hospitalization in three stages: Pre-hospitalization preparation, Hospitalization, Post-hospitalization transition care.

Here's what you do. Think of hospitalization in the following three phases and your outcome is likely to improve dramatically: pre-hospitalization preparation; the hospital stay itself; and post-hospitalization transition care. Your goals for the three phases: be prepared, create a healing attitude, and don't rebound back to the hospital. Did you know that one in five seniors who are hospitalized, treated, and released are back in the hospital within 30 days?[1] Stunning. To go through the shock and trauma associated with hospitalization, only to rebound back there again 20% of the time—that's a statistic an enabled Dr. You needs to avoid. Let's figure out how to do just that.

✚ PRE-HOSPITALIZATION: THE BIG PICTURE

How do you go about preparing for a hospitalization? It may be that a hospital stay is years away. It could be that you end up there after an unforeseen accident or health issue, which typically means an ambulance rushes you to the nearest facility. This begs the question: what brings us to the hospital in the first place?

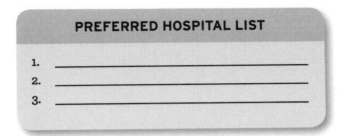

PREFERRED HOSPITAL LIST

1. _____
2. _____
3. _____

The two most common conditions for our age group are congestive heart failure and pneumonia. Interesting fact for you to know: over half of us will be admitted to the hospital through the doors of the emergency room. But often the incident that brings us there wasn't entirely unforeseen—so let's get planning.

First, just as there is variance in the quality of care delivered by physicians, not all hospitals are created equal, either. No doubt, some hospitals are "healthier" than others. But before I go on, let me start by thanking hospitals and their staffs. What would we do without these life-saving institutions of treatment, care, and healing? I shudder to think. Just try to imagine a vibrant, healthy, productive community without hospitals and their dedicated doctors, nurses, and health care professionals. These people are not only an integral part of your health and the health of your family, but they are essential to the growth and overall strength and vitality of your community.

It's with great affection that I recall my medical residency at the Hospital of the University of Pennsylvania. After years of classroom study, to finally be part of a team of professionals of such wide-reaching knowledge and passion was an inspiration. So much so that the experience is still vivid today, these many years later. The heck with the long hours and sleepless nights! Fatigue was no match for my youthful enthusiasm, and a desire to treat disease as a member of the healing arts.

Although my respect and admiration for hospitals has not waned, it is tempered by an important lesson that I've learned over the years. Despite the best intentions, the quality of care delivered from one hospital to another is inconsistent. Some professionals are better than others and some parts of the hospital are better than others. This variance can affect your health outcome, not to mention your safety and your financial security.

It's very important that Dr. You does a safety and quality check of the hospitals in your area. Just as you had to know your essential health numbers, you need to know your hospital's numbers. From outcomes on mortality rates to surgical infections to the safety record of the institution to patient satisfaction, there are many ways for Dr. You to get hospital-savvy.

Does this stuff really matter? It does—in fact, your health and life depend on it. For instance, an estimated 45% of patients don't receive care recommended by the best scientific evidence for their conditions, and 11% receive care that was not recommended or was harmful.[2]

HOSPITAL GUIDE

Questions to help you find the right hospital:

- Is the hospital accredited by The Joint Commission on Accreditation of Healthcare Organizations? See www.jointcommission.org.
- How does the hospital comply with recommended evidence-based treatment for your condition?
- Does the hospital have expertise for the condition that you need treated?
- Is the hospital included in your insurance plan's network?
- Does your doctor, specialist, or surgeon have admitting privileges at your hospital of choice?
- How safe is the hospital and how good are they at preventing infections?
- What's their performance record for patient re-admittance within 30 days of discharge?
- How does the hospital rate on "Patient's Experience of Care" measures, including pain management, communication about medicine, and discharge information?
- Would patients recommend their hospital to others?

Find answers to these questions and more at www.ahrq.gov, www.hospitalcompare.hhs.gov, and www.leapfroggroup.org.

Furthermore, did you know, for example, if you developed a health care-associated infection in the hospital that your average stay would extend from 5 days to 22 days?[3] That's an average of 19 more days in the hospital.

And then there's the tragic issue of hospital deaths due to preventable errors. In 2008, for Medicare beneficiaries alone, an average of 15,000 hospital patients a month experienced an adverse event that contributed to their death. Physician reviewers determined that 44% were clearly or likely preventable. That's 6,600 preventable deaths a month. Or the equivalent of 14.7 jet loads of Medicare beneficiaries dying from preventable hospital errors each month.[4] I'm not telling you this to make you fearful; I'm telling you this to convince you to engage Dr. You to make informed hospital choices.

✚ BECOMING HOSPITAL-SAVVY: START ONLINE

The steps for becoming hospital-savvy and choosing the right facility for you are as follows. One: get online and get your facts. Two: consult your doctor and health team. Three: talk to family, friends, trusted neighbors, co-workers, and community members. Four: make visits and phone calls.

Why don't more people do research and planning like this ahead of time? "I don't want to think about it," is a refrain I often hear, "because hospitals scare me."

What most often scares people? The fear of the unknown. Let's undo the unknown.

Start by firing up your computer, getting online, and learning about the quality of care delivered by hospitals. I've included a hospital guide to help you know what quality assurances you should be looking for when evaluating the choices.

A fabulous first stop is the Agency for Healthcare Research and Quality (AHRQ). A colleague and friend of mine, Carolyn Clancy, MD, is the director of the agency. She and her impressive team are on a mission to improve the quality of health care services, and to support research that helps folks like you and me make informed decisions.

SOURCES TO INFORM HOSPITAL CHOICES

- Get online and get your facts: Hospital Compare at www.hospitalcompare.hhs.gov, and Leapfrog at www.leapfroggroup.org
- Consult your doctor and health team
- Talk to family, friends, and trusted neighbors
- Make visits and phone calls

Their website, www.ahrq.gov, is actually your website—your tax dollars paid for it—and it's an information gold mine. For example, if you go into the sub-navigation under Consumers & Patients, and click Choosing Quality Care, there are a number of easy-to-understand tips featuring topics such as "Hospital Compare" and "Do Your Homework Before You Choose A Hospital."

One short column that particularly caught my eye is entitled *Does Your Hospital Do A Good Job?* It teaches, among other gems, that when patients are sent home from the hospital, only to be re-admitted again within the next 30 days, this re-admittance rate is one clue about the quality—or lack thereof—of care delivered.

Knowing that re-admission is a quality measure, you can further use the AHRQ website to link to the Hospital Compare tool at www.hospitalcompare.hhs.gov. Here you can check many important quality and safety performance measures for a hospital, including patient re-admission rates within 30 days. Low re-admission rates generally correlate with a higher quality of care, and to getting the right care at the right time using the latest evidence-based medicine.

As my friend Carolyn says, "Using Hospital Compare is like kicking the tires of your local hospital." I like that analogy. Hospitals are mysterious—sometimes secretive—places for most of us. Kicking the tires gives us a better sense of what to expect.

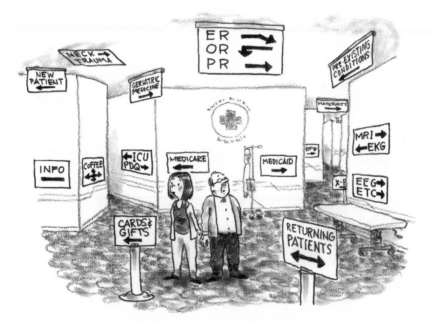

"Now I really feel sick."

Another valuable online source for making informed decisions about the quality and safety of hospitals is Leapfrog at www.leapfroggroup.org. A wise and prudent Dr. You needs to cross-check and validate findings by not relying solely on one source.

While you're online, you can also check the hospital websites. It will help you understand how they position themselves and if they specialize in certain areas like cardiac care, respiratory conditions, or diabetes, just to name a few.

Set aside a few hours this week to get online and do hospital research. It's amazing—not to mention fun—to Google things like "respiratory hospital Minneapolis." I found a hospital with 24-hour respiratory specialists for patients who need longer-term acute care. By typing in the condition you want to research, followed by the word "hospital" and your city, you'll make great progress toward the goal of becoming hospital-savvy.

The old world of a passive patient is gone. The new world of an active consumer of health care services is here. Tools like the ones you'll find at AHRQ and Leapfrog cast a bright, revealing light on once shadowy hospitals. We're entering the era of hospital accessibility, accountability, and a thing called transparency, which means there are fewer barriers blocking your view of the science-based facts.

✚ TALK TO DOCTORS AND NURSES

Now that your online searches have resulted in a few hospitals that look promising for your needs, talk to your doctor about them. Chances are that he or she will be able to offer further insight on your choices—possibly add to them. Your doctor will also be able to tell you what hospitals he or she has admitting privileges to. This is how your "comparison shopping" gets fine-tuned.

Don't stop there. Next, ask a nurse or two. Typically, if they don't have firsthand experience at a hospital, they have nurse friends working in the area who do. Collectively, through the nurse grapevine, they hear which hospitals are most committed to excellence and overall patient care.

✚ REACH OUT TO FAMILY AND FRIENDS

Family, friends, and neighbors are the next stop. Hopefully, by this point in your hospital homework, a few recommended locations are coming up over and over again. This kind of confirmation is a good sign, but you're not done yet.

Family and friends are especially valuable when it comes to issues of the patient experience with care. They've been to the hospital and have experienced things like how well the hospital team communicated and worked together, if pain was well managed, and if needs were promptly and respectfully met.

That said, don't be surprised if you run into a strong opinion in the friends-and-family step of the process. I remember a man telling me he was sure he went to the best hospital
in town. "Number five in the country!" he said, sure as can be.
After congratulating him I asked him how he was so sure. "Said
so in a magazine," he confidently answered. "The headline on
the cover was as big as a highway sign."

Just as we talked about when choosing a doctor, when
selecting a hospital that's right for you, be careful of the media's
hospital rankings and praises. Chances are the hospitals
splashed on the pages of magazines got there more by way of a
popularity contest or by placing advertisements than by credible
performance measures.

Also, please don't base your decision solely on hospital
hearsay, reputation, or sentimentality—"I'm going there now
because I went there as a child." And don't let laziness be the
deciding factor. Dig deeper. If someone hasn't already told you
this, let me be the first: you deserve the best—including the
best hospital for your needs.

✚ PHONE CALLS AND HOSPITAL VISITS

You're around the stretch turn and heading for the hospital-
savvy finish line. Lastly, it's time to get smarter by making a few
good old-fashioned phone calls.

Begin by asking if the hospital is in your insurance plan's network. If yes, go deeper. Tell the staff person that you're doing research on the best hospital for you. Ask to be connected to someone who can tell you what care the hospital specializes in.

You know that an informed Dr. You has to know his or her numbers. The same goes for a hospital: they have to know, and share, their numbers. Here's a real-life example: after years of living with a chronically achy, stiff shoulder, you're told by your doctor to get an MRI. The radiology report comes back indicating that you're a candidate for rotator cuff surgery. Your physician will likely mention a few hospitals whose services include such surgery, but it's up to you to do your homework. Now Dr. You needs to get smart about shoulder repair.

Go through your routine: go online to do your research. Ask around, starting with the doctor-recommended sources. Pick up the phone and call a few hospitals to find out how many such rotator cuff repair procedures they have done this year. Here's a tip: the respect with which your inquiry is treated on the phone is one indication of the care and quality of the facility. In more ways than one, a phone call can help in your decision of which facility is right for you, and which isn't.

Whenever you're visiting a hospital, have your "quality radar" up. Give the hospital environment the once-over with your eyes and nose. A well-maintained, spic-and-span appearance and a fresh, clean smell are good signs. Also pay attention to how the staff interacts and works together. Are they efficient, energetic, with a strong sense of camaraderie? And heck, are they friendly? Typically, a high degree of professionalism at all points of contact is part and parcel of a hospital that provides high-quality care.

"You don't have to be an old med student to know how good it feels to get homework done early."

Your homework is done! You don't have to be an old med student to know how good it feels to get homework done early. It's always smarter to research and choose a hospital preceding a need to go to the hospital, when things are calm and you're not in the throes of an emergency. This is the time to be deliberate, to get your facts lined up, and to think straight. Because when an emergency strikes, it's very hard to be wise and composed.

✚ WHAT "MINDSET" TO PACK FOR THE HOSPITAL

One important characteristic of the esteemed Dr. You is curiosity. Remember, a few chapters back, we learned that curiosity comes from the Latin *curiosus*, meaning to be diligent and careful and is akin to *cura*, which means care? Curiosity is how you get smarter. Curiosity is how you care. Curiosity is how to get the most out of the health care system by creating a short list of hospitals, and whittling them down to a fine few just right for you.

HAVING A GOOD HOSPITAL LIST PUTS YOU IN A HEALING STATE OF MIND

- Do your homework to find the best hospital for your and your condition
- Pack the right mindset for the hospital, including curiosity, a personal goal, and a positive attitude
- Identify your hospital advocate ("polite bulldog")
- "Teach back" important instructions
- Coordinate your care team and know who's in charge
- Organize discharge planning early, including setting up an appointment to see your primary care physician within 14 days
- Make a record of all new medications
- Assess the feasibility of home recovery and plan for health care assistance if necessary
- Ask your health team, family, and friends to wash their hands before touching you
- Focus on healing

Yes, preparation—there is no substitute. If illness or an accident strikes, you want to have done your homework so you can get to a hospital that fits your unique needs. Not only is that reassuring—helping you conserve precious energy—but you've also increased your chances for a best outcome. You've controlled what you can control, which should help give you peace

DR. YOU MEDICAL NOTE:

Pack the right mindset for the hospital: curiosity, personal goal, positive attitude.

of mind. I spoke with a surgeon friend of mine who confirmed that a less-agitated pre-operative patient is always desirable.

As a person prepares to go to the hospital, there are physical items to be packed in your hospital bag. But I want to talk about the mental aspect of preparing for the hospital. I call it, "what mindset to pack."

First, you have to pack the same curiosity that helped you find the right hospital in the first place. Be curious about your procedure. Understand it as best you can. Ask questions, and write down answers. Be curious about your recovery, your time frame, and your meds, to name a few. It's hard to focus on healing if you don't know what's healing, and how. The human body is an endless wonder. Be curious. It will help you heal.

Second, you have to pack a personal goal. It might have to do with length of stay. It might be paying extra attention so you have a solid grasp of the post-operative plan, and what you need to expect while recuperating back home. It might be to communicate more openly with your spouse—allowing yourself to be vulnerable and helped—letting your loved one know what you're feeling and what you need. Everyone's goal is different— that's what makes it a personal goal!

Third, you have to pack a positive attitude. As we talked about some pages back, being a "glass half full" person has been shown to improve health, and experts calculate it can extend lives as much as seven-plus years. Perhaps here's something you haven't considered: doctors and nurses are professionals, but they are human, after all. All other things being equal, whom do you think they will spend additional time and effort on, a positive patient or a negative patient?

So pack that positive attitude—right alongside your toothbrush and favorite pillow.

HOSPITALS ARE BIG. YOU ARE SMALL

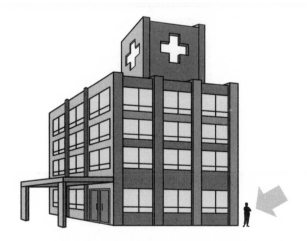

**Have a strong hospital advocate to keep
your care from falling through the cracks**

Oh, and I almost forgot one more very important item on your packing list. Chances are your primary care physician won't be your doctor in the hospital. And if you're in for an unscheduled, emergency procedure, your regular doctor won't even know you've been hospitalized. Your physician needs to be notified. Be sure to pack a note for someone to call or e-mail your primary care physician—be it the hospital or your family. Request that your regular doctor and your in-hospital physician (a doctor called a "hospitalist") have a peer-to-peer conversation about your care and follow-up treatment. Remember, the right hand needs to know what the left is doing. But you already knew that.

✚ THE PATIENT IS RESTING COMFORTABLY

We now move to the second of three phases of hospitalization, which is the hospital stay itself. Critical to the shortest, most successful stay in the hospital is a healing state of mind. Having a solid plan in place will make you more comfortable and promote healing.

If your hospitalization was predictable—say, a hip replacement surgery scheduled months in advance—planning comes easier. If an unforeseen emergency was the catalyst to your hospitalization, the thoroughness of your planning will quickly become evident.

DR. YOU MEDICAL NOTE:

A hospitalist specializes in care delivered inside a hospital. Hospitalists coordinate their work on behalf of primary care doctors who often confine their work to outside of the hospital.

Be sure to complete the simple list of your preferred hospitals. Share the list with your spouse, appropriate family member, or a trusted friend, depending on your situation. Whoever is going to be with you through your hospitalization—a person known as your "hospital advocate"—should have a copy of your list.

"Request that your regular doctor and hospitalist have a peer-to-peer conversation about your care and follow-up treatment."

Your hospital advocate is going to be at your side and on your side throughout your hospital stay. The quality to look for in a hospital advocate is what I call a "polite bulldog." Hospitals are big, busy places. You need someone making sure you're well cared for. A good advocate might have to follow the treating (or retreating) doctor to the back stairway to get a sufficient answer. A persistent, polite, firm temperament is what you're looking for in your advocate.

Chances are you're going to encounter some complicated medical instruction throughout this process. To aid recall, I want you to use a technique called "teaching back." This involves you and your advocate repeating back in your own words the doctors' decisions, instructions, and general concept of care. This type of attentiveness can keep important instructions from slipping through the cracks, which could prevent a less-than-optimal recovery, or even re-admittance to the hospital.

"Politely ask doctors and nurses who come into the room to treat you, 'Excuse me, have you washed your hands?'"

Before a hospital procedure, make sure Dr. You coordinates your care team. There may be a surgeon, a specialist, a hospitalist, nurses—so who's in charge? You need to ask. Who do you go to with questions or concerns? Find out who's leading your care team as early in the hospitalization as possible.

Counter to what you might think, early is also a good time to begin discharge planning. The hospital will have assigned

DR. YOU MEDICAL NOTE:

Don't forget to pack your primary care physician's phone number and email address so you can get your seven-day post-hospital appointment scheduled.

someone the responsibility to help you think about the recovery ahead.

Right off, ask the discharge planner to call or e-mail your primary care physician to notify him or her how the procedure went, and make an appointment for a post-hospital visit within seven to fourteen days. This is so important we'll talk about it again shortly when discussing transition care.

If recovery is planned at home, the discharge planner can help you understand what preparations need to be made. Who will be your home caregiver? Will you, for example, be returning home in a wheelchair? Can your home accommodate a wheelchair? Or might there be wound care or an around-the-clock schedule for medication? There's a medical term called "activities for daily living" (ADL) such as eating, bathing, grooming, toileting, and mobility. Is your caregiver capable—and willing—to assume these responsibilities, or will you need to bring health care assistance into the home? If you will be needing home care assistance, ask the discharge planner for recommended public and private sources. (We will be covering home health care in more detail shortly when we discuss transition care and your home safety net.)

Don't forget: the time to discuss these issues and assess real needs at home is early in the hospitalization, with your care team and discharge planner there, not a week later at 4 a.m. when you're alone with an emergency on your hands.

"Find out who's leading your hospital care team as early in the process as possible."

There's one more often-overlooked precaution you can take to keep yourself on the road to recovery. When doctors and nurses come into the room to treat you, ask them politely, "Excuse me, have you washed your hands?" Surveys show that patients are uncomfortable asking this question, but doctors and nurses don't mind being reminded of this simple but important precaution. Pose the same question when friends and family come to visit. Remember that frightening statistic about hospital infections and preventable death? It may be a bit awkward, but Dr. You needs to make sure that everyone treating and visiting you is as sanitary as can be.

Before leaving the hospital it's important that your hospitalist and your regular primary care doctor have a peer-to-peer discussion about your condition, including sharing the discharge summary, the new medication regimen, and how you are tolerating the new drugs. If there was difficulty scheduling your post-operative appointment with your regular doctor—for example, if the person answering the phone at the front desk said you couldn't get in for three weeks—many times this doctor-to-doctor discussion can fix that. Bottom line: chances of slipping

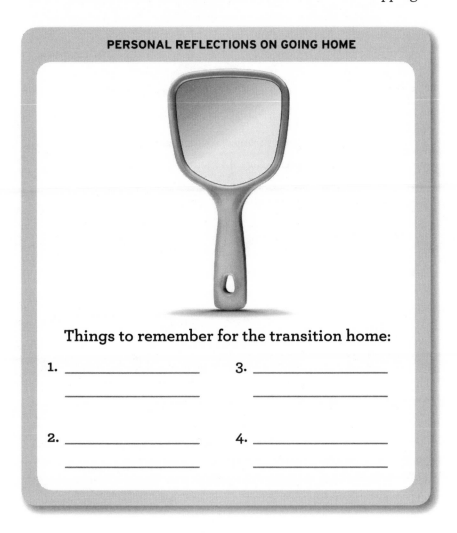

PERSONAL REFLECTIONS ON GOING HOME

Things to remember for the transition home:

1. _____   3. _____
   _____   _____

2. _____   4. _____
   _____   _____

ROLE OF THE CAREGIVER IN THE
THREE PHASES OF HOSPITALIZATION

Pre-hospitalization

- Know the patient's preferred hospitals and why
- Attend pre-op appointments
- Write down important instructions from the doctors
- To ensure a clear understanding was reached, "teach back" in your own words the doctor's decisions, instructions, and concept of care

Hospitalization

- Be a "polite bulldog" and advocate on the patient's behalf
- Be sure there is communication between the hospital doctor and the patient, and the hospital doctor and the primary care physician
- Know who's in charge of the hospital's care team
- Have a clear understanding of what to expect when the patient comes home
- Double-check that the primary care physician has been notified about the hospitalization
- Have the hospital help you set a follow-up appointment with the patient's primary care physician within seven to fourteen days

Post-hospitalization transition to home

- Coordinate care across different settings
- Recognize the vulnerability of the patient during transition—one in three are re-admitted to the hospital within 90 days
- Expect a phone call from the hospital within 24 or 48 hours after discharge to discuss the patient's medications, and any problems, questions or concerns. Call them if you don't receive this call
- Go to the follow-up appointment with the primary care physician
- Be patient, and get help so as to avoid caregiver burnout
- Find out about in-home health assistance at www.aoa.gov, www.eldercare.gov, or Google "elder home care pca"
- Help the patient to focus on healing

through the medical cracks and landing right back in the hospital are greatly reduced when the lines of communication from hospital and primary care physician are open and active.

✚ AVOIDING THE "REVOLVING DOOR"

Post-hospital transition care is such an important factor in a successful recovery, we need to devote a few more minutes to it. The first days out of the hospital are a particularly fragile and vulnerable time, especially for older patients. Done well, life can begin to transition back to normal—or better, if you had a successful hospital procedure. Done poorly, and your trip home won't last long. Here's what I mean.

As we saw earlier, according to Medicare data, about one in five senior citizens re-entered the hospital within a month of a discharge. Approximately one in three went back within 90 days. This is referred to as the "revolving door" of the hospital. The quality of transition care you receive after discharge can keep that door from spinning you back in.

Returning home is a challenging final step in the hospitalization process. There's a natural tendency to think, "Whew, we made it. The race is over." Subsequently, the family, and even the patient, can let their guards down. Attention everyone: the race isn't over! You're in the third, and in many ways, the hardest, stage.

DR. YOU MEDICAL NOTE:

When transitioning back to health at home, remember the three Cs: communication, coordination, and care.

First and foremost, be sure your home caregiver is in place. Oftentimes it's a spouse, family member, or trusted friend—perhaps all three working together.

Next, you and your primary caregiver should put together the month's calendar with important instructions, appointments, and goals. Put a big star next to the date that marks your follow-up appointment with the primary care physician. Don't forget to bring your brown bag of medicines with you to review with your doctor.

If there is no family caregiver available, or if extra help is needed, hopefully you spoke to the hospital discharge planner for leads. Furthermore, you can research public and private organizations for in-home health care help. Go to www. aoa.gov and www.eldercare.gov to learn about state and federal assistance programs. I also suggest you Google the Home Health Agency (HHA) and "elder home care pca." PCA is short for personal care aides. As the demand for home caregiving has skyrocketed in the past 10 years, many people have turned to personal care aides. These wonderful people can be a godsend to help with daily living activities like bathing and getting dressed. Also note, when you inquire among these groups, if they can't help, ask them to point you in a better direction. Another possibility: sometimes nurses or nursing students are looking to supplement their incomes; they can be good options as personal care aides.

When transitioning back to health at home, remember the three Cs: communication, coordination, and care. Dr. You should sit down with a family member and this book and talk about the best strategy for handling the entire hospitalization process. The best time to plan is sooner not later, when there isn't a pressing health issue requiring immediate hospitalization. Go over the role of a caregiver. Preparation is the best way to avoid getting stuck in the revolving door at the hospital.

✦ THE UNSUNG HERO: THE FAMILY CAREGIVER

A special note to all you who require caregivers after hospitalization and beyond: please be considerate of these amazing people. Oftentimes, upon returning from the hospital, you will be in pain or have some physical discomfort. It's easy to take out your suffering, frustrations, and even anger on those nearest, which is often your caregiver. Try your best to be as considerate as can be. Tell them "thank you" and acknowledge that they are doing a great job as they help you, rather than just accepting their help as an entitlement.

Provide honest, positive feedback. Tell your caregiver what's working, and what needs improvement. If possible, see if you can arrange for a break for them. There's a phenomenon known as caregiver burnout that we'll discuss in greater detail in the next section, but in short, fatigue from constant giving can become overwhelming. Show gratitude (make a card, use kind words), be positive and agreeable to your treatment, and try to provide an occasional break. These considerations—along with saying thank you so often you that you're on the verge of wearing it out—will go a long way toward avoiding caregiver burnout.

"Upon returning from the hospital, you'll likely be uncomfortable or in pain. It's easy to take out your suffering, frustrations, and even anger on those nearest, which is often your caregiver."

Your recovery will come with ups and downs. Your goal is to keep things as even keel as can be. Expect frustrating setbacks, try to take deep breaths, find your inner strength, and move forward with the kind assistance of your caregiver as the opportunity presents itself. Recovery is guided by the same principle that directs much of your behavior in this book—the solution lies in small steps. "The patient has to be patient," is a good motto to tuck away for a hospital stay. As you recover, find a bright penny every day. In time, your journey forward will have you feeling like a million bucks.

✚ SPECIAL NOTE TO CAREGIVERS

The goal is to help your loved one transition back to health and strength. The caregiver must brace for a rollercoaster ride. Some days will be better than others, more pain-free or painful than others, and more thankful or thankless than others.

There are a host of rather routine tasks that will need doing. Things like getting the mail, doing laundry, taking out the garbage, grocery shopping, picking up medications, and helping prepare meals, to name a few. You may also be responsible for some of the daily activities like bathing, grooming, and toileting. Not very glamorous work, but absolutely critical.

Oh, I almost forgot one other job that caregivers will have to do—this one for themselves: have their wings cleaned and pressed because caregivers truly are guardian angels. As the centerpiece of the transitional care team, they are the unsung heroes of health care.

Doctors and nurses tell me without exception that having a caregiver to coordinate the care from hospital to home is critical to a successful recovery. Without it, your chances of landing back in the hospital are frighteningly high. Family caregivers, you are the unsung heroes of the healing arts. Here's to singing your praises!

DOCTOR'S ORDERS
HOSPITALIZATION

- To get into a healing state of mind, do thorough hospital research.

- For best outcomes, approach hospitalization in three phases: Pre-hospitalization preparation, Hospitalization, Post-hospitalization transition care.

- Pack the right mindset for the hospital, including curiosity, a personal goal, and a positive attitude.

- Designate your hospital advocate: a "polite bulldog" who will be at your side and on your side throughout your hospital stay.

- Be sure your primary care physician is contacted about your hospitalization, preferably by your hospitalist (hospital doctor).

- Before being discharged, understand thoroughly the demands of home health care.

- Schedule and keep your follow-up appointment with your primary care physician within seven to fourteen days of hospitalization.

- Be appreciative of caregivers and watch for caregiver burnout.

Dr. You

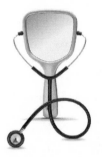

CHAPTER 8

THE RIGHT HEALTH INSURANCE PLAN

✚ A ROADMAP TO THE RIGHT HEALTH PLAN

Health insurance isn't a one-size-fits-all proposition—and to the surprise of many, that truism applies to both commercial insurance and Medicare plans. Another truism from previous chapters comes into play in this discussion about insurance plans, too. Namely, get involved and get smart. Your outcome can dramatically improve when you do your homework. There's nothing like the peace of mind of knowing that you've done your best and you and your loved ones are well-covered.

This book is written for a wide range of readers—from those in their middle fifties to those in their late eighties and beyond. Your health insurance options are equally diverse. There is something called commercial insurance, which is provided to people either through their work or they can purchase it on their own. There's Medicaid, which is health insurance for people with very low incomes. It's funded by both federal and state governments. And there's Medicare, which is federally funded health insurance for people 65 and older, and for certain younger individuals with disabilities.

> **"Whether you have insurance through your employer, individual insurance, Medicare, Medicaid, or no insurance, it's time to review the basics."**

Whether you have insurance through any of these channels, or no insurance, it's time to review the basics, know what's available, and make sure you're on the right track. I'm going to help you lay out an objective decision roadmap. This chapter, along with the many other resources at your disposal, can help you find the health insurance plan that's right for you.

✚ A QUICK REVIEW OF MEDICARE

We're going to look at Medicare insurance for a moment. For those of you not yet 65, consider this your warm-up exercise, so you're ready to jump into Medicare insurance with full confidence when the time comes.

How do you make the right choices? Your decision roadmap starts with a review of what's what.

I met a nice lady not long ago who calls Medicare "alphabet soup." She told me, "I can't keep my Part As from mixing up with my Part Cs and PDPs—which is which again?"

For her sake and yours, I will quickly highlight the key differences. For a deeper study, I suggest you go to medicare.gov. It's filled with great information—from the basics to the detailed—plus links and contact information for help. I also suggest you Google "health insurance companies." You'll find that company websites can be outstanding resources for everyone looking for insurance.

In the end, we all need a helping hand to get us through the insurance choices. The companies that you'll find on your Internet search and medicare.gov have customer support representatives who can expertly clear the way and help you with your decision roadmap. Okay, now on to alphabet soup.

Part A. This is your hospital insurance. It helps cover inpatient care in hospitals, skilled nursing facilities, hospice, and home health care services. Most people with Medicare insurance don't pay a monthly premium for Part A. We talked about hospitalization in the last chapter. In the next chapters, we'll discuss life at home, or in other residences should health issues bring you there. Part A insurance plays a role in that discussion.

DR. YOU MEDICAL NOTE:

You can qualify for Medicare before age 65 if you have a qualifying disability.

Part B. This covers medically necessary services like doctor visits, outpatient care, home health services, and some preventive services. If you have Medicare, take out your card and check to see if you have Part B. Typically you pay a monthly premium to Social Security.

RESOURCES FOR GETTING SMART ON INSURANCE PLANS

- Look at health insurance company websites, visit medicare.gov, and consult with SHIP
- Talk to friends, family, trusted community members, and co-workers
- Go to your local bookstore or library
- If employed, talk to the benefits or HR manager or company owner

Part C. Also know as a Medicare Advantage plan. It's a plan choice that you may have as part of Medicare. Sometimes you'll hear the term "MA" used for a Medicare Advantage plan. Part C or MA plans are offered by private companies approved by Medicare. If you join an MA plan, it includes all your Part A (hospital insurance) and Part B (medical insurance) coverage, and most plans include Part D (prescription drug) coverage. It may offer extra coverage for important services such as vision, hearing, dental, and health and wellness programs. Medicare pays a fixed amount for your care to the companies offering Medicare Advantage plans. Medicare sets the rules that these companies must follow, but different out-of-pocket costs and different rules for services can apply. For instance, what is the referral policy to see a specialist, and can you see only doctors who are in-network? These are the kinds of questions you'll want to look for and ask about as you find the plan that fits you best.

Part D. This is prescription drug coverage. Although it is a Part of Medicare, it's only available through private companies. There are two ways to get Medicare drug coverage: Medicare Prescription Drug plans ("PDPs") and Medicare Advantage plans. The cost of each plan and the drug coverage can vary. Medicare Advantage Plans with prescription drug coverage are sometimes called "MA-PDs." You must have Part A and Part B to join a Medicare Advantage plan.

If you join a Medicare Prescription Drug plan or a Medicare Advantage plan, you still need to enroll in Part A and Part B. Medicare needs to know that you're enrolled even though you will be getting your benefits through a private company.

Medicare Supplement plans. These plans are not a "Part" of Medicare, but are often confused as such. A Medicare Supplement plan (sometimes called "Med Supp") helps you pay for out-of-pocket costs like deductibles and copays that

Medicare doesn't cover. Think of it this way: Medicare pays first, and then your plan "supplements" the other payments. A common mistake is confusing the Medicare Advantage plans that we just talked about with a supplemental plan. See the chart just below as a good starting point for understanding the distinction between Medicare Supplement plans and Medicare Advantage plans. The chart compares things like restrictions on choosing doctors and hospitals, access to specialists without referrals, flexibility to make changes anytime throughout the year, and more.

	MEDICARE SUPPLEMENT INSURANCE PLANS	MEDICARE ADVANTAGE PLANS
Choice	Select your own doctors and hospitals, as long as they accept Medicare patients.	You may be required to use network doctors and hospitals.
Access	See specialists without referrals.	You may need referrals and may be required to use network specialists.
Freedom	No network restrictions. Coverage goes with you, across the United States.	You may have network restrictions. Emergency care only for travel within the United States.
Flexibility	You can switch to another available Medicare supplement plan at any time.	Generally, there are specific periods during the year when you can switch to another Medicare Advantage Plan.
Cost	Monthly plan premiums in addition to Part B, with limited out-of-pocket costs.	Low or no monthly plan premiums, in addition to Part B, with deductibles, co-insurance and co-payments when you use services.
Prescription drug coverage	None. Consider purchasing a Medicare Part D plan.	This coverage may or may not be included, depending on the plan you choose.

Change in plans? Between October 15 and December 7, you can join, switch, or drop a Medicare drug plan (Part D). The same is true for Medicare Advantage plans (Part C). Also, in this timeframe, you can drop your Medicare Advantage plan and go back to Original Medicare (Part A & B), or opt to add a Medicare Supplemental plan to Original Medicare. Your change will take effect on January 1 of the following year as long as the plan gets your request by December 7.

> **"Line up a nice day with a trip to your local bookstore or library and get a book on health insurance plans."**

I can't disagree with the woman who said that's a lot of alphabet soup. But as we learned from our wise mothers, soup can be good for health. It takes time and questions to understand this, but you're not alone. Learn more at the insurance company websites and at medicare.gov. When you're there, look for contact information to connect you to people with answers. Remember, you're first eligible for Medicare during the seven-month period that begins three months before you turn 65, includes the month you turn 65, and ends three months after the month you turn 65. Also remember that you can qualify for Medicare before age 65 if you have a qualifying disability.

✚ KNOW WHAT PLANS ARE AVAILABLE

What specific health insurance plans are available to you? It's time to put on your research hat, pull up to a computer, and start investigating your choices—beginning with visiting some of the old familiar places.

I'm hoping you've been to medicare.gov to learn more about the Parts of Medicare. That website is a treasure trove of information about what plans are available, too. Did you find any consumer assistance contacts, including the dedicated Medicare helpline?

Also look at the insurance company websites. You'll be able to click through to product offerings there. They too have dedicated professionals available to answer your questions.

If you want more detail about available plans, certainly there are many good books about Medicare and pre-Medicare insurance. Line up a nice day with a trip to your local bookstore or library and see what you can learn.

Again, whether you're looking to find out more about Medicare or pre-Medicare insurance plans, talk to friends, family, and co-workers. Ask about their personal insurance experiences. Are they happy with their plan and insurance company, or are they shopping around? Discussion can help demystify insurance and put the plan choices in real-life terms. Don't, however, just listen to one opinion and be done. Have multiple points of contact to draw upon.

If you're employed, bring a few questions (and maybe a cup of coffee) to your benefits or HR manager. Oftentimes, he or she is a good friend to have and can really help. If it's a smaller company, talk with the owner. If you're retiring soon, ask if the employer offers retiree coverage. If retiree coverage does exist, ask about cost, coverage, and what happens if you choose to insure another way.

If you're self-employed, there are a number of plans you can find using many of the sources already mentioned. Did you know you may be able to lower your insurance costs through a membership organization? Getting your insurance through, for example, unions, alumni, and professional organizations such as your local chamber of commerce may be a smart option. Hey, I have an idea. Now that I've written this book, I will Google "writer, health insurance membership benefits." Wow! The top three hits give me options on health care plans that leverage the power of a group.

Ask your primary care physician, too. He or she may have an opinion about insurance plans based on your health, and on experiences gathered from other patients. They will also be able to tell you if they are "in-network" (a participating physician) for particular plans and if they are a Medicaid provider.

When you're gathering your facts about plans, do a little homework around the insurance companies, too. Ask yourself what you've heard about their reputation. Dig a little deeper:

how's their financial stability? How many members do they have? More members generally translate into more price stability because the risk is spread out across a wider group—especially in Medicare supplement plans.

Finally, for information about Medicaid eligibility, coverage, and services, contact your local Medicaid office by going to www.benefits.gov and typing "[your state] Medicaid" into the search bar.

HEALTH PLAN CHECKLIST

Ask about coverage of these services and costs
- Inpatient hospital services
- Outpatient surgery
- Emergency room care
- Pre-existing conditions
- Work-related injuries
- Prescriptions
- Medical tests, x-rays
- Preventive care, routine check-ups
- Physical or speech therapy
- Hospice care
- Choice of doctors
- Mental health care
- Immunizations
- Physician office visits
- Monthly/annual costs
- Individual premium/monthly
- Family premium/monthly
- Individual deductible/year for medical care
- Family deductible/year for prescription drugs

✚ LOOK IN THE MIRROR TO ASSESS YOUR NEEDS

By now, Dr. You has gotten very good at looking in the mirror and being honest about what barriers are between you and better health. When it comes to your health insurance plan, a similar self-examination is key to making the most fitting choice.

Understanding your expected needs from the medical system is the place to start.

What care do you foresee requiring, and what plan addresses those needs? Meanwhile, your insurance provider will be equally interested in your medical needs, so they can align you with the best choice.

Take a moment. Have a good look in the mirror. First, how's your health? Are you generally in good health, or do you have a number of chronic conditions?

Next, let's look at your prescription medications. Get your complete drug list together, along with how regularly you're taking them. On the bottom of your drug list, note how much you're spending on prescription meds.

What about your health team? What doctors do you have, where, and for what type of care? Ask yourself, "Am I open to seeing a new doctor?" Changing plans could mean changing your doctor, but many plans have large networks so oftentimes you'll be able to keep your doctor. That will be one of the questions you'll want to ask.

How much do you travel? Is it mostly inside the U.S. or do you often travel abroad?

If you're 65-plus, are you eligible for coverage besides Medicare? You may want to keep some of that coverage.

How much did you spend on medical care last year? That total can help you estimate next year's cost.

And finally, how does health care fit into your budget? Will you need financial assistance to afford monthly premiums? If you think you might qualify for assistance, apply as soon as possible. It can take several months to process an application and determine eligibility.

"Changing plans could mean changing your doctor. That will be one of the questions you'll want to ask."

✚ FIND THE PLAN THAT FITS

Much is changing in the world of health insurance, and your needs may be changing too. With those needs in mind, you're armed to find the best plan to fit you and your resources. Go back to the insurance websites and medicare.gov. Remember, you'll be looking for a specific plan, and a specific company handling the plan.

DR. YOU MEDICAL NOTE:

Medicare choices and guidelines for Parts A, B, C, and D are not the same state to state, or even county to county. The first thing a provider will ask for is your ZIP code.

To narrow your search, you can contact the insurance company's consumer representatives using the information provided on their websites. Lay out your general needs. See what products they suggest for you. I've included a checklist of 19 specific services and coverage issues that you can ask about. Do this with each company on your list. Comparison shop as you go, until you find the right fit.

Many insurance companies, as well as medicare.gov, have a plan finder tool on their websites that can help you see what plans align with your needs. The process begins with a ZIP code because the specifics of a plan often change by state—even by county.

Another must-see source to assist you is SHIP, short for State Health Insurance Assistance Plan. SHIP is a free, impartial Medicare counseling service, including Medicare Advantage (Part C) and Medicare Prescription Drugs (Part D) plans, Medicare Supplement plans, Long-Term Care financing plans, Medicaid, and other low-income assistance programs.

SHIP's mission is to help you get the most value for your health care dollar. What's more, they can refer you to other appropriate agencies for your needs. Every state has SHIP, but note, the name may change. For example, Ohio's state service is called OSHIP. You can find more at shiptalk.org.

"If there's a way financially to consider long-term care insurance, I urge you to look into it further."

You may be looking for some very particular services in your plan. Some plans and companies, for example, offer a nurse line as a contact point for questions, or even care managers who will monitor health and help coordinate care. Other particular services you may be looking for could include dental, hearing, or vision coverage. When comparing plans, inquire about special services like these and broader issues such as: how many doctors and hospitals does the company contract with? And do they have resources to help you find the specific doctors and hospitals that are really good at what they do?

Just as some doctors and hospitals are better than others, some insurance companies and plans are better than others. Do the homework you've gotten so good at. You know the routine: get your facts online and from friends, understand your unique needs, make some phone calls, do your comparison shopping, and find a plan that fits.

These are patient-centric times. Insurance companies are working very hard to align you with the right product, and are busy competing for your business. Take advantage of your leverage!

FIVE TIPS YOU WON'T WANT TO FORGET

- You're not "stuck" with your choice. In fact, about 5-10% of Medicare enrollees switch plans annually. You can do so between October 15 and December 7
- Enroll as soon as you are eligible. If you wait, you may have fewer options and you may have to pay more
- Where you live makes a difference. Your choice of plans and the cost will vary based on where you live
- Understand what you will be paying
- Don't be afraid to ask for help

✚ LONG-TERM CARE INSURANCE

Long-term care (LTC) insurance can help protect you and your family from the potentially catastrophic financial burden associated with caring for a loved one's chronic illness or disability. This insurance can help cover the significant costs of in-home care for services such as visiting nurses, home health aides, home-delivered meals, and respite services for caregivers, to name a few. If instead, your loved one needs to reside in an assisted living facility or a nursing home, LTC insurance could help cover those skyrocketing costs.

Long-term care insurance is expensive, and for many, not financially feasible. But if there is a way to absorb it into your budget, I urge you to look into it further. As we will discuss in the upcoming chapters, the demands of caregiving—physical, emotional, and financial—are tremendous. Long-term care insurance could be one way to lessen those burdens.

DOCTOR'S ORDERS
THE RIGHT HEALTH INSURANCE PLAN

- Remember, beginning in 2011, the annual open enrollment period for making changes to your Medicare insurance plan is from October 15 to December 7.

- You're not "stuck" with your choice. In fact, about 5-10% of Medicare enrollees switch plans annually.

- Create a decision roadmap: know what options are available, know your medical needs, and find the right plan.

- Get smart on choosing an insurance plan by visiting the insurance companies' websites, going to medicare.gov, reading books, and talking with friends.

- Learn your Parts. Part A: hospital insurance. Part B: medical insurance. Part C: Medicare Advantage. Part D: prescription drugs.

- Ask friends, family, and co-workers about their insurance plans, and their level of value and satisfaction.

- Be sure to consult SHIP (State Health Insurance Assistance Plan) for free, impartial Medicare plan counseling services.

- For Medicaid eligibility and services, contact your local office by going to www.benefits.gov and typing "[your state] Medicaid" into the search bar.

Dr. You

SECTION 3
HOME AND FAMILY

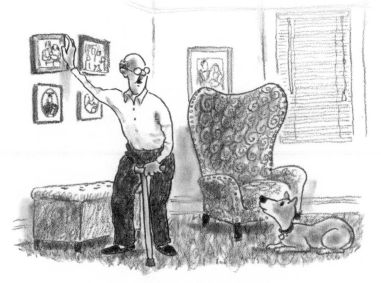

"Not to worry, boy.
Life is full of little adjustments."

We've come a long way, dear Reader. We began with under-standing disease and its prevention or minimization. Moved to health-enhancing adjustments in diet, physical activity, and life-style. Next you mastered the steps to choosing the right doctor, hospital, and insurance plan. And you gained a much greater awareness of the goals for your medications—as well as their potential dangers.

"When it comes to the quality and longevity of your life, home and family are about as important as it gets."

Now we're going to bring it all home. Literally. To wherever you happen to live. To whatever family you have—near or far—to share your life with. And let me be clear, I include friends in this group, because friends are often family, too.

Home and family—how I love those words. When it comes to the quality and longevity of your life, home and family are about as important as it gets. We will discuss why in the coming chapters.

I hope you're at home reading right now. Even more, I hope you're in your favorite chair, surrounded by a feeling of peace that you hadn't even noticed until I just mentioned it. Do you feel it? How do you tap into that peace more often, more deeply, and draw greater health from this place called home?

We will soon see how home can be much more than a structure with a roof, four walls, windows, and a few squeaky doors. Home can become a part—or an extension—of the health care system, helping you to be as healthy as can be.

Beyond home, we will talk about family, and how family—even if they're time zones away—can help support your health. We'll also see how your family, friends, and community can be woven into a safety net of relationships. My friends, prepare to become a beautiful weaver of safety nets.

And finally, we'll talk about sitting in that favorite chair of yours, closing this book, and contemplating the fullness of life. The fruits of those thoughts will help you in the book's last chapter on end of life planning. I want to be clear: end of life planning is not and should not be a somber experience, nor is it a statement proclaiming that you're near death. To the contrary, end of life planning is a celebration of the fullness of life that brought you to this moment, and it is a look forward to plan how to get the most out of the years ahead. It's a guiding light for you and your loved ones.

Change is happening all around us—and *to* us—as we age. We have to make peace with that change, and then Dr. You has to manage it to the best of your abilities.

This last section of the book is about taking control, and it is about vulnerability. Ironically, those words are not opposites. In fact, it is the acceptance of our vulnerability that makes us less vulnerable. We become stronger through ourselves, through our surroundings, and through others. And with this strength we manage change.

> **"It is when we accept our vulnerability that we become less vulnerable, and become stronger through ourselves, through our surroundings, and through others."**

I think you're going to really like what's ahead. Starting with an honest look-in-the-mirror inventory of your home's safety. As you'll learn, some home hazards are as obvious as an electrical cord stretched across the middle of floor. And others are as invisible as dust mites in a pillow.

CHAPTERS IN THIS SECTION:

9. Healthy Home

10. Creating Your Personal Safety Net

11. End of Life Planning

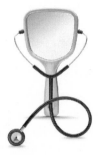

CHAPTER 9

MAKING HOME HEALTHIER

✚ HOW HOME SHOULD FEEL

Be it ever so humble, there's no place like home. I wish I were the first to pen that sentiment. Truer words have never been written.

Home is the place you've worked for your whole life. On a practical level, it's built to maintain and protect your health—call it your port in the storm. More so, home is the place where you are most comfortable. You feel safe there—happy and settled and surrounded by good memories and possessions. Home is a place of peace and quiet, and as we age, we tend to spend more time there. You should feel capable and in control in your home. As you will soon see, home is the center of your safety net. A cozy, peaceful feeling should reside there with you.

For some of you, a loved one may reside there, too. Perhaps a spouse or a partner of many years—or of a few—where you share one of the greatest of all gifts: companionship. For others, perhaps by choice or circumstance, you live alone. We all have different needs and preferences when it comes to our living spaces, and how crowded they're meant to be. But please, if you do live alone, do not let it be an excuse to become isolated. No matter our living situation, we all need to connect with others in order to be healthy.

Now although home can be a place of deep contentment, if you're not careful, it can be a place of dangerous health hazards, too. Hazards that can land you in the hospital.

Let me help you become more aware of your living space. Our goal: make it as safe and healthy as can be. My career working in and with the health care system has given me an insider's view of just what home hazards send seniors to the hospital over and over and over again. It's time to slow this unnecessary parade of older adults to the emergency room. It begins with a home inventory. Let's find the trouble spots around the house that you can easily correct and make safer on your own, and discover those that you may need a little help with.

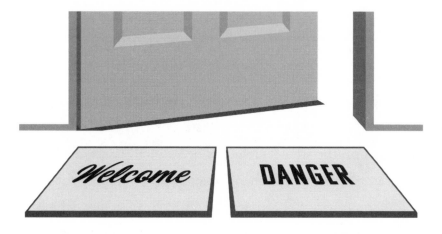

How many health hazards exist inside your home?

✚ HOME SWEET HOME?

You've been doing a fantastic job of holding up the mirror and facing what you can do to have a healthier lifestyle, and how you can improve the medical decisions you make. Now I'd like you to hold that mirror up inside your house and make an honest room-to-room assessment of the safety of your living space. Just as your body is an environment to protect your health, so too is your home an environment to protect and promote your physical, mental, and spiritual well-being.

Before any of us can make meaningful change—be it in ourselves or in our homes—we have to recognize that something needs changing in the first place. In the case of your home, that's not so easy, because in many cases you've been living with the hazard for years without incident. What's more, as you've aged, you've changed, not least of all physically.

So here's the question: as you've aged, has your home changed to meet your evolving heath needs? A little turned up carpet on the step, which only occasionally caused a harmless stumble, can now launch a major fall. A slippery shower stall with no handrail can now lead to a hip fracture, which can lead to a cascade of health issues that you don't want to imagine.

Dr. You, it's time to give your house a check-up. That's right. Just as you need an annual check-up, so too do your living quarters. Think of it as preventive medicine in the form of a room-to-room inspection. Let's discover and eliminate potential problems before they cause injury or aggravate a disease or injury. It's time to look at your house in a different light. Namely, the bright light of an examination room.

THREE OF THE MOST COMMON CAUSES OF FALLS

- Rugs
- Electrical cords
- Pets

✚ LITTLE THINGS THAT CAUSE BIG THINGS

Look for the little things around the house because they can cause big things. Let me make this point more real by sharing the stories of two different women with surprisingly similar fates. Rather than use their real names, I'll use nicknames to emphasize my point. And hopefully, it will help you remember these hidden dangers as well.

FALL PREVENTION CHECKLIST: YOUR HOME

- Be attentive!
- Clear walking pathways of papers, books, shoes, and other clutter
- Tack, double-stick tape, or otherwise secure rugs and electrical cords
- Install railings on stairways
- Make sure your home is well-lit, including nightlights
- Install grab handles in the shower, tub, and toilet area if needed
- Put non-slip mats in the tub or shower
- Check your sidewalks and driveway for cracks and uneven areas
- Use non-slip floor wax and wipe up spills immediately
- Stay off ladders and chairs for hard-to-reach areas
- Have your vision and hearing checked
- Check your medications; some can affect balance
- Do your balance and strength exercises
- Wear flat shoes with rubber soles around the house
- If at risk, find the appropriate fall alert device to monitor your safety

---

The first woman I will affectionately call Ms. Three Things At Once (know anyone who fits that description?). She's very active, in her middle 50s, and always has one too many things on her dance card—typically running behind as a result. One afternoon, Ms. Three Things At Once was (1) talking on her cell phone, (2) quickly getting dinner ready, and (3) letting the dog outside when she tripped over the dog at the door. The poor woman somersaulted down the steps, fracturing her collarbone.

> **"Remember Ms. Three Things at Once, Mrs. Ruby Red Throw Rug, and Mr. Night Tripper. Be careful not to end up like they did."**

The second woman I will call Mrs. Ruby Red Throw Rug. Her agility and mobility were slowly on the decline due to arthritis, but not to a degree where anyone was overly concerned. One of the centerpieces of her home was a favorite possession: a glorious, hand-hooked, ruby-red throw rug that had accompanied her on every move from young motherhood through empty-nesting. One evening, while hurrying to answer the phone, she caught her toe on the upturned lip of that throw rug, giving new meaning to the words "throw rug." She was rushed to the hospital with a broken hip, which in turn led to complications with her arthritis and respiratory issues because of the associated long, sedentary recovery time.

Right now you might be thinking, "Not me. I don't need to worry about falls."

Really? Let me give you an idea what kind of epidemic falls have become. I just looked at a survey which showed that more than one-third of adults 65 or older had fallen in the last year.[1] Furthermore, falls are the leading cause of fatal and nonfatal injuries in this age group.

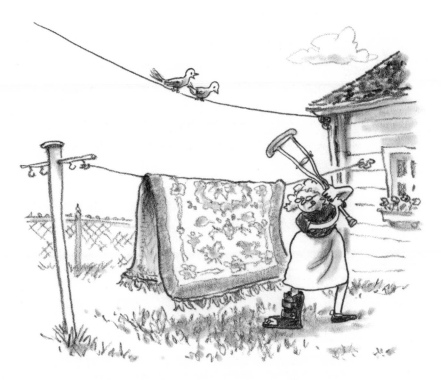

"It tripped her. So it's getting a spanking."

DR. YOU MEDICAL NOTE:

Over 90% of hip fractures are caused by falling. And one out of five hip fracture patients die within a year of their injury.

Another report showed that falling and being at risk of falling had a stronger influence on quality of life than many common chronic health conditions (such as diabetes, hypertension, arthritis, and respiratory conditions), from both a physical and mental health standpoint.[2] This is why you need to make your home a safer environment to move around in. Unquestionably, the risk of falls is a danger you must address.

Let's look at this a little closer. Over 90% of hip fractures are caused by falling. And one out of five hip fracture patients die within a year of their injury.[3] Dear Reader, this potential killer is oftentimes preventable just by doing little things around the house.

Have a look around your house. Can you guess what three of the most common causes of falls might be? There were clues in the first two stories. They are: rugs, electrical cords, and pets. Go around your rooms on a "little things" search. This is no snipe hunt, believe me.

Your to-do list should start with things like tacking down or removing rugs. Re-route and properly fasten electrical cords away from high-traffic areas. And make sure your in-home walkways are free of shoes, books, magazines, or other house-hold clutter that you can trip over. Also, please don't walk around your home in socks; they slip on far too many surfaces. Have a comfortable pair of rubber-soled shoes for getting around in. Take a look at the included fall prevention checklist and use it as you survey your house.

Another key to fall prevention are the physical activities we discussed earlier in the book—remember? "Six Butterflies Sipping Cocoa" (SBSC): stretch, balance, strength, and cardio. Include this in your fall prevention routine—especially the balance and strength exercises. They will truly increase your safety at home.

I talked to a man not long ago who told me he never gave any of this fall-prevention stuff a second thought until... I'll call my friend Mr. Night Tripper. He was making his usual late-night visit to the bathroom when he tripped over an exten-sion cord that was running an extra fan in the bedroom. Luck-ily, he got out of it with nothing more than an unsightly bruise. That was his wake-up call, so to speak.

So when you see shoes left out where they are a tripping hazard, or a rug that is not secured down on a rubber, no-slip pad (usually found where rugs are sold, and at "big box" hard-ware stores), or a stool left out just waiting to trip you up, think about Ms. Three Things at Once, Mrs. Ruby Red Throw Rug, and Mr. Night Tripper. Which one is most like you? Then do what it takes to avoid the pain and suffering they went through. Remember, all it takes is a few little things to cause a big problem. Or to avoid it.

✚ CLEAN IS HEALTHY

Beyond preventing falls, what's one of the most important precautions we can take to make the home safer? The answer is so obvious that you're probably looking at it the moment you lower your book. Can you guess? The answer is to keep your house clean.

Dirt, dust mites, pet dander, bacteria, mold, mildew and the like are unhealthy, unwanted houseguests. They trigger allergies, reactions, and sickness that can worsen chronic illness—especially, for example, respiratory disease like asthma. Did you know that about 1 in 12 people suffer from asthma?[4] If that doesn't include you, chances are it could include a friend coming over to visit, a son or daughter, or even the little lungs of a grandchild.

My philosophy: the older you get, the cleaner your home needs to be. Vacuum often. Get new pillows and be sure to wash bedding weekly in hot water, including the blankets. And don't bring food into the bedroom. It invites pests and other unhealthy visitors to follow in for the crumbs.

Keep countertops and food prep areas clean. Don't let dishes pile up in and around the sink. Use a dehumidifier to reduce humidity to below 50% and be sure to fix leaky pipes, dripping faucets, and other sources of moisture. Scrub moldy surfaces using a cleaner with bleach, and replace moldy shower curtains. Replace your furnace filters, and have ductwork cleaned. If there are some tasks you can't do by yourself, we'll be talking soon about how to get help from others. Also, take care

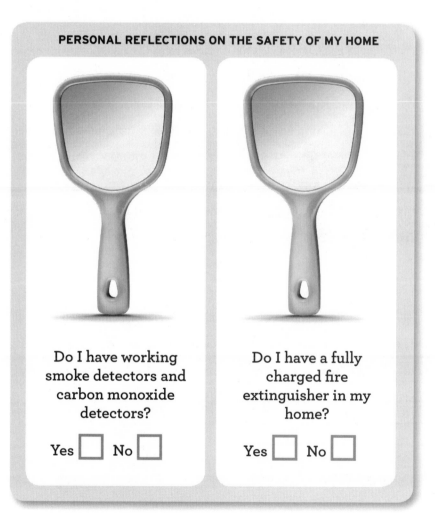

PERSONAL REFLECTIONS ON THE SAFETY OF MY HOME

Do I have working smoke detectors and carbon monoxide detectors?

Yes ☐ No ☐

Do I have a fully charged fire extinguisher in my home?

Yes ☐ No ☐

One of the most important precautions you can take to make your home safe and healthy is to keep it clean.

to be vigilant about pest and rodent control. And of course, no smoking in the house—or anywhere else, for that matter!

CREATE YOUR QUIET, HEALTHY SPACE

Once your home is clean, there's one other thing I'd like you to do around the house for your health. Maybe you've already done so, but if not, I want you to establish your quiet space, a place of peace, where you can escape for a moment and ponder the many wonderful things in life. You've worked so hard, accomplished so much, and come so far; you deserve a place that's all your own where you can reflect, restore, and renew. It's a little like rebooting your computer when overuse has the system locked up.

Remember when you were a child? Did you have a safe, hidden place you'd crawl into where you could get away from it all? I did. The fact is we still need a quiet, healthy space where we can think and be at peace. Maybe it's a cozy chair with a window view—there may be a nearby photograph of family or a memento from a wonderful trip. Is that your favorite music playing I hear?

To tell the truth, that description is pretty much what my healthy quiet space is like. No TV. No loud distractions. Just a quiet, stress-free place that's all mine. Why do we need such a place? Stress and chronic anxiety are major contributors to illness. Stress and chronic anxiety rob you of energy. Energy is the stuff of life. A quiet, peaceful place recharges you.

Create your own quiet, healthy space. Find a better frame of mind. Feel the good. It will help keep you young, like a child in a secret, out-of-the-way spot.

"Create your own quiet, healthy space where you can reflect, restore, and renew."

✚ DR. YOU AND THE HOME COMPUTER

A key component of homes today is the computer. In many ways, it's the newest window in your home—that is, along with the Internet, it's your window to the world, one which connects you to so much information and so many friends and loved ones.

Thanks to the computer—and smartphones and tablet computers—70% of American homes are able to access the Internet. This means that most of the Dr. Yous out there now have your own personal medical library right at your fingertips.

DR. YOU MEDICAL NOTE:

With the Internet and a home computer, you can build your personal health library.

Throughout this book I have referenced websites that are chock-full of simple tips and strategies to help you help yourself in the pursuit of better health. Those websites are just some of the exciting ways that Dr. You can use the computer to improve health. Just be aware that there are medical websites that aren't reputable. Stick to the ones I've mentioned, or those recommended by your physician, your health plan, or medical associations.

Did you know that many of today's computers come with a tiny camera installed in them? Look up there near the top of your screen. You may see a little camera embedded there. This enables the computer to go beyond just being your health library. You can reach out to friends and family to make free video calls where you can talk and see one another on screen. Yes, I said free. (If you don't have a camera on your computer, you can attach one very affordably.)

What you need to do is Google an amazing technology called Skype. It's so easy—and it's free. By installing the application on your computer, you can use Skype to connect with people almost as if they were in the room with you, as long as they have Skype on their end, too. If your computer doesn't have a camera, you can make computer-to-computer voice-only calls using Skype, too. Skype is a fun, healthy way to use your home computer to stay better connected with those who want to hear about your experiences and share theirs.

How about Facebook? Are you a registered user? I know, I know, it's just for kids, right? Wrong. It's amazing how many older adults are using Facebook to engage with the world beyond their four walls. Did you know that about 25% of Facebook users are 50-plus? Hey, it's free and it's fun and it's a way to reach out and get more social—which, as we talked about earlier, can improve the quality and longevity of your life. If for no other reason, get on Facebook so you can communicate with the nearly impossible-to-reach grandkids in your life.

Bottom line: don't hog all of you to yourself. Share on Facebook. It's fun. And speaking of fun, while you're at the computer, there are also numerous games and brainteasers you can play online to keep mentally sharp, too.

✚ HOW YOUR HOME CAN BECOME AN EXTENSION OF THE HEALTH CARE SYSTEM

Here's a final thought on how your home can positively impact your health. Certainly the Internet, along with your home computer, is changing how modern health care information is being disbursed. But did you also know that there are many medical devices that offer life-changing, life-sustaining possibilities right in the comfort of your home?

What I tell people is that thanks to these in-home devices, your home can become an extension of the medical care system, monitoring or treating an illness, and even transmitting data back to your medical team. Not only is this technology impressive, it's becoming very user-friendly, too.

Rather than a technical description, let's make this concept real by using a case that was recently brought to my attention. A woman suffered congestive heart failure when her high blood pressure went undetected and untreated. This episode damaged her heart muscle, weakening its ability to pump blood out to the rest of her body. This in turn caused fluids to build up, indicated by weight gain. All in all, it was a life-threatening situation.

Luckily for the woman, she had previously done her homework and found a hospital that had an outstanding safety rating and was recognized for excellence in cardiac care. Guess what? Once she was stabilized, her care team sent her home where they were confident she would recover nicely. But they didn't send her home alone. A critical part of her recovery and ongoing treatment was the careful monitoring of her weight, so she and her care team would know if fluids were reaching dangerously high levels. All this was done at home!

DR. YOU MEDICAL NOTE:

In-home medical device technology can now link you to your health team, making your home an extension of the medical care system.

She had an electronic scale that connected to her home phone and transmitted critical vital data like weight gain to her care team. This way even subtle changes could be detected and communicated. She called this device her "electronic nurse." This connectivity kept her actively involved in her daily treatment and kept her home, where she wanted to be.

This story is an example of a health care win-win that can often lead to fewer trips back to the emergency room and a decrease in re-admissions to the hospital. That can save lives as well as your hard-earned money. Now do you see what I mean when I say these medical devices can make your home an extension of the medical system? Pretty cool.

Similarly, there are sensors that can be used to alert others in case of a fall. I know what you're thinking, dear Reader. You're thinking about those "I've fallen and I can't get up" jokes or t-shirts that poke fun at the old television commercial. Let me tell you, the subject of falls is no joking matter. I have had an experience in my family where someone who had fallen couldn't be heard calling for help—and chances are you know of someone, too. Why do we wait for a tragedy to sound our wake-up call? A visit to the emergency room—or worse—is a very large price to pay for trying to outwait an accident.

As a result of the lessons I've learned, I bought my mother an alert device for Christmas. Undoubtedly, it's one of the best presents I've ever given. It's hard for me to say who's more comforted by the device: my mother or me and the rest of the family knowing it's there if she needs it. Does it slow her down? Ha! I'd say it's been quite the opposite.

If you or a loved one is at risk of falling, or spend a good deal of time alone, look into alert devices. They can simply clip on a wrist or be worn on a pendant. Rather than seeing them as a burden or a tether, they can greatly increase your independence and confidence because you and your loved ones now have a plan in place should a fall occur. That's called controlling what you can control, one of the primary themes of this book, right?

Maybe your response is, "Phooey, Dr. Reed. I might be getting a little shaky, but falling has never been a problem for me." So it has never happened before, huh? Exactly! That is the very definition of an emergency—an unhealthy, unplanned accident. This book is about avoiding dangers before they become emergencies. When you can't predict it, you need to try to prevent it.

So talk to your doctor about what you can do at home, and how some of the devices in the rapidly growing field of biometrics and telemedicine can help you. There are a number of life-changing, lifesaving devices available that equip your home to deal with the demands of aging so you can be as independent and worry-free as safely possible.

One final thought. Remember how we discussed the home computer cameras that allow you to have video calls with other members of your family or friends at their computers? Well that's just the tip of the iceberg. We're on the cusp of technology that lets you handle some of your medical appointments this way, too. Imagine not needing to go across town to see your doctor, not sitting in the waiting room, but having a face-to-face consultation with your physician as you sit in front of your computer and he in front of his. All from the comfort of your own home.

We are living in revolutionary times in the world of home-based medical technology. From vast medical websites to pocket-sized in-home health monitoring tools, I urge you to integrate these breakthroughs into your life. Embrace the advancements! I want Dr. You on the cutting edge, benefiting from all the exciting things here today and to come tomorrow.

DOCTOR'S ORDERS
MAKING HOME HEALTHIER ℞

- Make your home a place where you are surrounded by healthy contentment.

- Recognize your vulnerabilities. Ironically, it will make you less vulnerable and better able to mange changes in your life.

- Be attentive to the biggest causes of falls, including rugs, electrical cords, and pets.

- Don't underestimate the dangers of falls. Falls cause 90% of hip fractures, and one out of five hip fracture patients dies within a year of injury.

- Keep your home clean. It is one of the most important precautions you can take to keep your home safe and healthy.

- Inside your home, create your own quiet, healthy space where you can reflect, restore, and renew.

- Use your computer and the Internet to build a personal health library that you can consult often.

- Consult your doctor about in-home medical devices that can help you live more vigorously and independently.

Dr. You

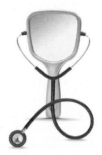

CHAPTER 10

CREATING YOUR PERSONAL SAFETY NET

✚ YOU'VE EARNED YOUR SAFETY NET

We can learn so much from a simple net. Think about it. Thin strands of rope—individually not particularly strong—but when laid side-by-side and woven together, the whole becomes stronger than the individual strands.

Think also about how each strand of rope has to "reach out" to the next strand to bring strength to the whole. This weaving together, these interconnections, is what makes a net sound and strong. Truly, this is the perfect metaphor for how home, family, friends, community, and public and private services can be intertwined to create your custom safety net.

"By weaving together relationships between home, family, friends, community, and public and private services, you can create your personal safety net."

"Who needs a safety net?" you might scoff. "I'm no circus performer."

Well it may be that you didn't run away with the circus, but life can be a high-wire act, especially as we age. Things get a bit precarious, and that's what safety nets are made for.

It gets back to my earlier point about vulnerability. Many of us are reluctant to acknowledge that we can't do it all ourselves. You need to understand and accept your vulnerability—doing so is part of the wisdom of aging. People will be strong for you, just as you have been—and will continue to be—strong for them.

Maybe your youthful bravado assures you that you can be an island. Or perhaps you were hurt in a way that caused you to vow not to trust again. It's time to put those thoughts aside. They're not the answer. Relationships are the answer. Your life is as strong as your relationships, or as frail.

Let's look at another definition of vulnerable: to be open or exposed. As you age, better health requires that you are open. Open to ideas as well as love. Let me tell you something that I hope will sink in. When doctors are diagnosing the possibility of depression, a key question we ask a person is, "Can you give <u>and</u> receive love?" Please forgive this inelegant metaphor, but your pipeline has to be open both ways. Give. Receive. Got it?

You've given so much. Changed so many diapers. Mopped so many runny noses. You've laundered, cooked, transported, and provided for family for most of your life. Part of what you need to learn from this chapter is that it is okay to take a little back. You deserve it. You need to be open to receiving the love and support of others.

We all become stronger by weaving others into our lives—just as the net is stronger than the individual strands of rope. When you get your safety net under you it's an inspirational feeling. Interconnectivity gives you such strength. So let's get at it.

THE ROWS IN YOUR SAFETY NET

Ready to weave? Not so fast. First, you have to assess the size of the safety net required for your very unique needs.

The process begins when Dr. You looks in the mirror and does a personal inventory. How much help do you need? Just a little now and then? Or conversely, maybe your health situation calls for a full-time caregiver. Or perhaps you are a full-time caregiver for a loved one, and you're at your wit's end desperately needing a break. The point is, each of us is so different, and so too are our safety nets.

What keeps a person from taking a personal inventory and identifying their needs? You'd be surprised by the folks I meet and the barriers they have erected. There are all kinds of people in this world, but here are a few of the types that I meet over and over again (maybe you'll recognize one or two): The all-powerful-me type. We talked about them. They are lone eagles, too proud to ask for help. The I'm-not-worthy type. The I-don't-want-to-be-a-burden type. The too-shy-to-ask-for-help

CREATING YOUR SAFETY NET

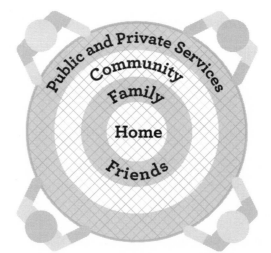

type. The I'm-all-alone type. And the head-buried-in-the-sand type. Honestly, I'm most like the I-don't-want-to-be-a-burden type. But I'm taking some of my own medicine and working on it. I'm getting better, which is all this book asks of its readers. It's important to know that whatever type any of us are, there's a safety net we can weave to help.

> **"Let family and friends be strong for you. You have been strong for them."**

It all begins in the center with your home. That's why we worked so hard in the last chapter to make your home as healthy as can be.

The next row out is family and friends. Let them love and help you. When you do, that's you reaching and weaving the center and the first row together.

The next row after that is community, including neighbors and volunteers from your place of worship, civic associations, social organizations, and so on. Again, by reaching out to include them, your safety net gets broader and stronger. Adding this row can also take some of the strain off you and your family and friends. Or, if you have little or no family to help, this row brings in an important new dimension to your safety net.

DR. YOU MEDICAL NOTE:

Recent statistics show that 25% of the U.S. workforce juggles work and caring for a loved one.

The next row out after community includes public and private services. Public services are often provided by state and federal government agencies and non-profit organizations. And private services are offered by individuals and companies who specialize in in-home health care. Again, it's important that you reach out to this row of resources when necessary.

Do this and you will have a strong, diverse safety net to call on in times of need. For example, let's say you need transportation to the grocery store to shop for some of the delicious, healthy food and beverages we've discussed. Some of you may need to use a state-provided service to help you find that transportation. Others of you might get that transportation right from the center of your net, from your spouse or a relative who lives with you. In my hometown there's a non-profit agency that shops for seniors and delivers the food right to your kitchen counters. It all depends on your personal situation and your personal safety net.

What's most important is that you understand the concept of a safety net—and see its value and necessity. Don't be an I'm-all-alone type. You don't have to be alone. Don't be an I-don't-want-to-be-a-burden type. You're not a burden. How do I know? Look at the rows in your net. You have given to those rows for your whole life. Heck, you helped make them strong in the first place. Home, family, friends, community, and public and private services—those rows radiating out are there not only to support you, but to nourish you.

Your safety net will help you stay healthy as can be, or to return to health when illness occurs. It's proof, once and for all, that no one is an island. No one should be. And no one has to be. That's nice to know, isn't it?

"A caregiver and a loved one need to sit down together and look at caregiver information together, so everyone goes into these changes with eyes wide open."

✚ HOME: THE CENTER OF YOUR SAFETY NET

Now I'm going to talk about home as the center of your safety net. I hope the previous chapter gave you plenty of ideas on how to make your home a healthier, more nourishing place.

For each of us, home looks different. You might live alone, or you could be raising a whirling dervish of a grandchild. You could be living with one of your children, or with a spouse.

DR. YOU MEDICAL NOTE:

Caregivers spend on average about 20 hours a week giving care.

Men, let me pause for a moment to talk about our spouses. My career in health care has taught me one thing for sure: women are the chief health officers of the family. They may badger and pester us about our health, but truth be told, we're darn lucky that they do. Keep up the good work, ladies. If I had to offer an educated guess I'd say that women make 70% of the health care decisions for the home. Oftentimes, that's a lot of thankless work.

Guys, we need to step up. It's not fair to put that burden on our spouses, especially as they age. With this book as your guide, you can now become a much more active part of your heath care team, starting right at home.

As the calendar years flip by, a time may come when you need more care at home than you can handle alone, or that your wife or partner can provide. That's when it's time to call on the next row out in our safety net.

✚ FAMILY AND FRIENDS: THE FIRST ROW OUT

Think about family. What is it? In a literal sense, it's those we are connected to by birth, marriage, or adoption. But a more complete definition would include the enduring sense of roots, traditions, and togetherness. (Yes, even despite our family squabbles.)

Remember the TV show *The Waltons*? Remember how the show signed off each week with the scene of the family farmhouse at nightfall? Today it might seem a little corny, but that image so ideally captured the essence of family that we still remember it these many years later: the closeness of family, all within earshot, each saying goodnight, bedroom after bedroom.

It makes me think about what this scene might mean on a deeper level. The farmhouse is home, and family is family, but perhaps nightfall is symbolic of aging. As we move beyond our twilight into our later years, we need more than ever to be close to family. Family is the light in the bedroom window; it's the nearby voice that says goodnight and confirms you're not alone.

Others may think it's just an image from a television show. I will admit, programs like *The Waltons* or the *The Cosby Show* with the Huxtables did present idealistic family scenarios—and I certainly hope you don't get depressed watching these idyllic TV families that few of us could ever hope to replicate in real life. But underneath the stage lights and the makeup and the rehearsed lines, there was a real truth: family connections do make us better, stronger human beings—even with the imperfections that all families have.

Maybe your relationship with your family is exemplary, perhaps not. No matter what, now's the time to tighten up your family around you, to reach out to strengthen those connections—or perhaps, to overcome long-endured differences. Reach out. Mend your net as you mend your fences. It could be the real value of family is right there in front of your nose and all you had to do was reach for it.

You need to talk openly about aging, and what effect it might have on the family as a whole. If you haven't already, talk about roles and responsibilities that different family members or friends are comfortable with. Who could be a primary caregiver? Who is better at assisting? If you're dealing with a serious health issue, is there someone who best understands the illness and the care demands that come with it?

Every person and every family is different when it comes to expectations about involvement with their parents' or their elders' later years of life. A person's culture and the way he or she grew up will influence their decisions. Some family members might say it's their duty. Some might say it's their pleasure. Some might say it's out of the question. You need to have this important discussion so you can weave your safety net accordingly.

I have a Navajo friend, for example, who will do almost anything to keep his elderly parents at home, caring for them, for as long as possible. This tradition is an unwavering part of his culture and personal philosophy. But again, every culture and family is different.

TEN TIPS FOR FAMILY CAREGIVERS

1. Choose to take charge of your life, and don't let your loved one's illness or disability always take center stage

2. Remember to be good to yourself. Love, honor, and value yourself. You're doing a very hard job and you deserve some quality time, just for you

3. Watch out for signs of depression, and don't delay in getting professional help when you need it

4. When people offer to help, accept the offer and suggest specific things that they can do

5. Educate yourself about your loved one's condition. Information is empowering

6. There's a difference between caring and doing. Be open to technologies and ideas that promote your loved one's independence

7. Trust your instincts. Most of the time they'll lead you in the right direction

8. Grieve for your losses, and then allow yourself to dream new dreams

9. Stand up for your rights as a caregiver and a citizen

10. Seek support from other caregivers. There is great strength in knowing you are not alone

Contributed by the National Family Caregivers Association

I'm sensitive to the fact that, for numerous reasons, many of you don't have family to call on. If so, the first row of your safety net often includes a good friend or friends who could step in and provide care. As many of us know, friends can be a second family. Throughout my career, I have witnessed inspirational examples of caregiving by best friends and even groups of friends who created a rotating schedule of care for a loved one.

Ultimately, your unique needs and situation will determine how much support comes from the first row of your safety net. It could be an occasional visit, to check in on you. It could be driving you to doctor appointments and being there to write down important instructions. Or it could be a much more demanding commitment.

Caregiver involvement, especially long-term involvement, depends not only on the health condition of the loved one, but also on the availability of the caregiver. Recent statistics show that 57% of caregivers are in the workforce, adding significantly to their responsibilities.[1]

Let's talk about what it takes to become a long-term caregiver for a family member or loved one, and how to accomplish it in the healthiest way possible for everyone involved.

✚ LONG-TERM FAMILY CAREGIVING

We touched earlier on caregivers and the critical role they play during and after a hospitalization. The context for that discussion was more short-term: getting a loved one through hospitalization and recovery.

Now let's look at the challenging subject of long-term family caregiving. In your specific situation, you may be a caregiver, or you may be the one receiving the care. One thing is true no mater what: this is a partnership. Caregiving is not all give or all receive—especially long-term caregiving. It is a team concept—just as the success of your physician relationship and hospital stays relies on team.

Good caregiving should begin with a heart-to-heart conversation between all parties involved. Does everyone fully understand the illness and the care it will require? Is the home equipped for such care? Can the long-term caregiver commit the time and energy that this role demands? Does it involve a move for a family member or parent? Can the caregiver still manage her or his direct family responsibilities beyond those needed by their parent or relative?

Statistics show that millions of caregivers have both childcare and eldercare responsibilities. To handle these additional responsibilities, 20% of caregivers have to take a leave of absence from work—and almost 10% have to quit their job.[2] Obviously, the decision to become a long-term caregiver is a big one.

What is a potential caregiver to do? Once you understand the illness and the necessary care, start by assessing your skills specific to that care. Every situation is unique. The caregiver

> **DR. YOU MEDICAL NOTE:**
>
> Ask yourself, "Am I equipped and is the home equipped to handle this illness?" Also consult your family and the loved one's physician.

may have to assist in the activities of daily living such as feeding, bathing, grooming, and toileting. Physically demanding duties might be required for mobility, such as lifting a person in and out of bed. Or maybe the caregiving will require constant vigilance of a loved one's safety issues caused by a disease such as Alzheimer's. A long-term caregiver has to start by sizing up the needs and then honestly evaluating one's personal ability to meet those needs.

Furthermore, every long-term caregiver should build a care team. No one should try to shoulder the burden alone. There are a number of tips and checklists for caregivers and care receivers that we'll look at shortly.

Should you decide to be a long-term caregiver, I want to emphasize one point in particular: get regular breaks and keep yourself healthy. You cannot be a source of health if in so doing your health fails. I've included a set of tips on that subject.

What I've learned is that once the requirements of care have been assessed, and a support team has been assembled, the long-term caregiver needs to learn how to succeed in her or his new role. And because this is a two-way street, the loved one needs to learn how to *accept* caregiving, too. Thank goodness for some amazing websites on this topic offering tools like checklists to prepare for caregiving, training manuals, and videos created by experts and caregivers themselves—there are even message boards where those receiving care or providing care can go for answers and support. You and your caregiver need to sit down and look at these websites together, so everyone goes into these changes with eyes wide open.

HOW CAREGIVERS HELP THEMSELVES

- Exercise. Add much-needed physical activity to your daily routine so you don't sacrifice your health for the health of another

- Eat properly. Don't neglect your nutritional needs

- Make and keep your own doctor appointments. Again, be sure to protect your health

- Keep a journal or diary. This way you can better assess how things are changing over time

- Pursue hobbies. Make sure that you're still doing things that bring you joy

- Blow off steam. It's okay to step away and take a break when you need to

- Tap into others in the safety net. Don't try to do it all alone. Dole out some of the responsibility

- Accept the help of others. Trust their sincerity and take them up on their offer to help

- Join a caregivers support group. Great comfort comes from talking with people who "get it"

- Practice relaxation techniques. Release the stress of caregiving

- Use the websites provided here for information and support

You can start at any of the websites I've listed here. At www.aarp.org, type the words "getting started as a caregiver" into their search bar. It will provide you with great reading and videos on the subject. See also the Family Caregiver Alliance at www.caregiver.org, plus www.caregiving.org and www.fullcir-clecare.org. Each of these is a marvelous resource, providing insights and tips on getting started, building a support network, what kind of costs are associated with caregiving, a checklist of questions to ask an aging loved one, and so much more.

✛ FAMILY CAREGIVER BURNOUT AND ELDER ABUSE

Speaking frankly, caregiver burnout and elder abuse are difficult issues to discuss. But they need to be addressed because certain situations can lead to behavior that can't be safely ignored.

Sometimes, as demands remain great over an extended period of time, pressures can intensify and caregivers can suffer from burnout. Caregiver burnout can lead to depression and other health and behavior issues. That's when help from other family members, community volunteers, or public and private services needs to be brought in. There are times when we simply must reach out and get the next rows of the safety net involved.

Caregivers, hear this: what you're doing is extremely difficult work. There is no disgrace in asking for assistance. If you feel yourself nearing a snapping point, walk away, take deep breaths, cool down, and find some additional help. That's your responsibility. Know when to seek help and then get it.

How do you know where that snapping point may be? Begin by trusting your instincts. Nobody knows you like you. You can also Google something called the Zarit Burden Scale to help assess if you're in danger of a collapse. I really like this scale. It's an eye-opening 22-question "interview" about how you feel, your stress and anger levels, and how your health is being impacted, to name a few. There are no right or wrong answers; you just circle the number that best describes your feelings. Then share your results with you primary care physician. If he or she has experience in geriatrics, chances are they have this test in their office.

Things can escalate. Sometimes a caregiver can go from being frustrated to overwhelmed to angry to finally becoming neglectful or abusive. Abuse is totally unacceptable, as well as being against the law. If you or someone you know is in immediate danger, call 911 or the local police. If the threat is less immediate, log on to National Adult Protective Services Association at www.apsnetwork.org and click "Report Abuse." Another source for elder abuse is the National Center on Elder Abuse at www.ncea.aoa.gov, look for the help hotline. You can also call 1-800-677-1116 on weekdays.

DR. YOU MEDICAL NOTE:

The Zarit Burden Scale is used to help caregivers assess if they're in danger of a collapse. Google "Zarit" for a 22-question interview.

I'm going to share a heartbreaking story with you. Uncomfortable as it may be, part of our author-reader relationship calls for honest disclosure, even in difficult situations.

Not long ago, as part of my mission to improve how health care is being delivered across the nation, I was on a phone call between an elderly woman and a nurse who helps coordinate her care. The elderly woman lives with her daughter. The nurse, as part of her job, was talking with the woman about her medications, her diet, and her general health. With permission, I was able to listen in. As the conversation went on, it became obvious from the elderly woman's halting words that something was wrong in the home. The nurse and I began to sense that the woman was in an unhealthy, unsafe environment, but she was reluctant to talk about it. The conversation went like this:

"Mrs. Jones," the nurse asked, "are you getting enough to eat?"

There was a pause. "Sometimes," she said.

The nurse then asked, "Does your daughter cook for you?"

The elderly woman said, "Sometimes."

Then she asked, "Does your daughter ever yell at you?"

And after a long pause the answer was "yes."

And then the elderly woman was asked, "Does your daughter ever hit you?"

And the only reply that came across the line was silence. So the question was asked again. "Mrs. Jones, does your daughter ever hit you?"

And after a very long pause, very softly, the woman said, "Yes."

Tens of thousands of elderly Americans are abused every year, often by their caregivers. It might be a daughter or son, it could be a spouse, or it could be someone hired to be a caregiver. This cannot be allowed. Your dignity is something that should never be stripped away by any other human being. If you or someone you know is the victim of elder abuse, you need to contact adult protective services. Go to www.apsnetwork.org to find out how to report abuse. This means any kind of abuse: it could be physical abuse, emotional, financial, or even sexual abuse.

To be in need of care does not diminish your value, your beauty, or your rights. This is nothing to sweep under the rug. An abusive situation needs to be dealt with right now. So contact adult protective services. You deserve to be treated with respect and dignity.

✚ ADDING COMMUNITY TO YOUR SAFETY NET

After family and friends, the next row out in your safety net is community. Community includes neighbors and volunteers from churches, synagogues, mosques, temples, civic groups, and the like. If you just give them a chance, there are numerous opportunities to weave these people into your life. More often than not, they are thrilled to help.

Chances are that you yourself know the deep satisfaction that comes from volunteering and helping others. There's a beautiful phrase written by Robert Greenleaf that I've always

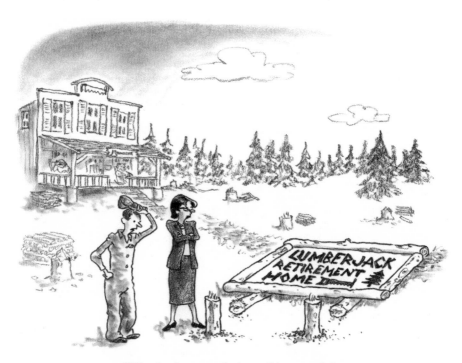

"That's the second time this month."

held close to my heart: *Serving each other, the more able and the less able serving each other, is the rock upon which a great society is built.* It's in our core as human beings to give of ourselves. And you also need to be willing to receive. It's how our world thrives.

Let me tell you about a volunteer named Jim. Jim's a retired electrical engineer who's never met a faulty lamp he can't rewire, a garage door opener he can't install, or a leaky faucet he can't fix. He's a magician with tools. Jim is retired, but guess what? His skills aren't. He enjoys helping others. It is his way of staying sharp, sharing his skills, and giving back for all he's been given.

Remember when we were going through the home safety checklist? Chances are there were things on the list that, unless you're like Jim, you can't do by yourself. It could be climbing on a ladder and replacing batteries in your smoke detectors. Or something more involved like installing a grab bar in your shower. One way to accomplish these important safety tasks is to ask a neighbor if they know anyone who could help. They might surprise you with their handiness, or know someone who fits the bill. Other options are to ask at your place of worship or a civic organization. Many of us don't need to learn to become Mr. or Mrs. Fix-it. We only need to learn to ask for help. And by accepting help, you're letting another show off what they're good at, and that gives them worth and value.

Getting back to Jim. He says he'd much rather show up at a person's house with a few tools in hand to make a home safer than show up at the hospital with flowers in hand because something unsafe didn't get fixed. I think that's a very good way of putting it.

Community can help in so many other ways, too. Perhaps it's shopping for groceries together. Or someone can help you with heavy lifting around the house. Or snow removal, or yard work. Think about what you need help with. Make a list. Then get some help from the next row out in your safety net. Who knows—you might just make a new friend or renew an old relationship in the process, too.

✚ BROADENING THE SAFETY NET TO INCLUDE PUBLIC AND PRIVATE SERVICES

There are numerous public and private organizations that can provide us with vital services as we age.

To locate government-sponsored services, one of the first resources to use is a group called the Administration on Aging, found at www.aoa.gov. Their mission is to develop a comprehensive, coordinated, and cost-effective system of home- and community-based services that help elderly individuals maintain their health and independence. They can help you find local services in your area to assist with things like grocery shopping, meal delivery, home cleaning, transportation, in-home health services, and more. Also check out The Area Agency on Aging found at www.services4aging.org. Folks, these are important resources. Check them out and bookmark them on your computer.

> ### TIPS FOR CHOOSING AN INDEPENDENT LIVING FACILITY OR NURSING HOME
>
> - Independent living community: www.alfa.org
> - Nursing home checklist: www.medicare.gov/NHCompare

You may also be eligible for caregiver services provided through your health insurance. Be sure to call and inquire about your options. Good insurance companies work hard to help you maximize your health and independence. When you are talking to various agencies, be sure to ask what services are or are not covered by private insurance, Medicare, Medicaid, or VA benefits if you qualify for them. Ask your insurance company, too. They want you to stay healthy; be sure to tap into them and see if they can help.

Another great resource that you'll want to weave into your safety net is the Eldercare Locator, a public service of the Administration on Aging. Go to www.eldercare.gov and connect to extremely helpful community services in your area. For example, you may need help with Alzheimer's, or home repair and modification, or contact information on in-home care services. The Eldercare Locator can help you with that and so much more. Don't be too proud or too shy to reach out. Remember, many of these services are government-funded—so all your working life you've been contributing to making them strong. Think of it as a bank account that you've been paying into for years. Now it's time to make a withdrawal.

By weaving public services into your safety net, you can take some of the strain off the other rows. As we talked about before, the whole of the net is stronger than the individual strands. If you can't connect to these websites from home, go to the library and log on there. Or look in the phone book.

The best safety nets often extend wider and wider yet. For some, this might require weaving in private care resources. We talked earlier about in-home personal care aides (PCAs). Again, I suggest that you start by Googling "pca services [your state]," or "In-home health care [your state]." You can also try www.care.com. What I expect will happen is that once you start digging, you will find the right service and provider for you. The key is you have to begin digging.

One final but important note: as you reach beyond family and friends for in-home health care, you have to be sure you're mentally prepared to bring someone new into your home. The difficulty of this decision varies depending on the person or the family. Of course you'll want to check that the in-home health

DR. YOU MEDICAL NOTE:

Before reaching out for professional in-home health care, be sure you're mentally prepared to bring someone new into your home.

professional is insured and bonded, but beyond the proper certification, this is an emotional decision. Take some alone time and some family time to consider it. There are a number of wonderful professionals available to you. You also need to be ready for them.

✚ WHERE'S THE RIGHT PLACE TO LIVE?

As a person's health and ability to live independently wanes, the choices of where to live for the next stage of life are many. I always tell people facing this decision that the goal is to live in a place that offers the greatest independence for your level of functioning. Please remember, dear Reader, this important point: having independence and living independently are not necessarily the same thing. In fact, many people find greater independence in living situations outside the home. The key is to know your options.

Your options range from long-term in-home care, senior housing with services, small group homes for seniors, assisted living communities with varying levels of care, nursing facilities that provide immediate levels of care, to nursing home care.

> **"When talking to various agencies and businesses about in-home care, ask what services are or are not covered by private insurance, Medicare, or Medicaid."**

What you need to do is contact these facilities to see what's right for your very personal needs. There are many ways to find locations in your area, including contacting your local Area Agency on Aging at www.seniorslist.com, and using the website from our last section: www.eldercare.gov.

As you have done throughout this book, Dr. You has to return to the mirror and ask the tough question: is home really the right place for me now, as it was before? Start by looking around. How easily accessible are the bedrooms and bathrooms in your current home? What about the laundry room? Are you still in good enough health to manage the upkeep around the house? Are you in an area that's safe for walking? Are you near public transportation, a grocery store, and your place of worship? What about friends and family—are they nearby? The answer might be yes, the answer might be no.

What about affordability? Can you manage the mortgage payments, taxes, and upkeep? Some people who are dealing with affordability issues are turning to the possibility of shared

DR. YOU MEDICAL NOTE:

All in-home health professionals should be certified, bonded, and insured.

housing. Go to www.nationalsharedhousing.org and see if that option makes sense for you.

"Your goal is to live in a place that offers the greatest independence for your level of functioning."

If you do have a long-term caregiver, and you do agree that you want to stay at home, consult with your doctor. It is amazing how homes today can be set up with the equipment necessary to be well cared for there. I am not telling you that this is the right option; I'm saying it's one of the options to consider.

If the demands and seriousness of the illness have advanced beyond the capacity of your in-home caregivers, then it is time to look at other options. We've gone through a list of choices. What do you look for in, say, an assisted living community or a nursing home? There are comprehensive overviews and checklists that I want you to look at so you're well prepared. For independent living communities go to www.alfa.org. For nursing homes go to www.medicare.gov/NHCompare. Of course, you and your family need to visit the locations and talk with key staff members.

This may be the right time to have your safety net extend out to private sources. For some, finding new living arrangements is exactly the right decision to manage increasing health needs. If so, be assured: there are many older adults who transition wonderfully, finding friends, peace of mind, and joy awaiting them as they move into a new phase in life.

DOCTOR'S ORDERS
CREATING YOUR
PERSONAL SAFETY NET

- Weave your safety net of family and friends, community, and public and private services.

- Be willing to accept help from neighbors and area volunteers. Part of our value as a human being is realized by serving others.

- A long-term caregiver has to start by sizing up a loved one's needs and then honestly asking: "Can I meet those needs?"

- Watch for early signs of caregiver burnout and take precautions not to let your health suffer.

- If you or someone you know is in immediate danger from elder abuse, call 911. If the threat is less immediate, go to National Adult Protective Services Association at www.apsnetwork.org and click "Report Abuse."

- When talking to various agencies and businesses about in-home care, ask what services are or are not covered by private insurance, Medicare, or Medicaid.

- All in-home health professionals should be certified, bonded, and insured.

- When considering where to live, your goal is to find the place that offers you the greatest independence for your level of functioning.

Dr. You

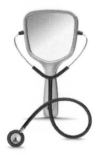

CHAPTER 11

END OF LIFE PLANNING

✚ PUTTING YOUR LIFE PUZZLE TOGETHER

As Dr. You certainly realizes, at some point we have to have a frank talk about how to prepare for and manage our end of life decisions. What are our goals? How do we want to be cared for? Where do we want to be? How can we be sure our wishes are upheld?

Throughout the journey of this book, we've never shied away from honest, sometimes difficult topics—that's part of the author-reader relationship that was set forth in the first pages.

Death is a natural part of life, yet as much as we know that to be true, the thought of it is often frightening. But like most other things in life, with planning comes comfort.

You can hardly turn a page in this book where we haven't discussed the importance of pushing aside the barriers and taking control of your health to the best of your ability. This central theme certainly doesn't diminish as we approach the end of life—if anything, this last phase of life is when we need to remove the remaining barriers and take control all the more.

> **"Eliminate the mental clutter of daily concerns to find the peace and contentment that comes with end of life planning."**

When we are terminally ill or threatened by a sudden catastrophic event, life-sustaining and life-ending decisions will be made. You want to be sure that your wishes are followed. Not the doctor's. Not the hospital's. Not the state's. Not the wishes of the most forceful member of your family. None of these. Your wishes. Your plan. We all need to approach end of life with the peace of mind that our plan and our wishes will be honored. After all, it is your life.

When I informed my editors that I intended to conclude my book with this topic, guess what? They were against it. They thought it would be "a downer."

I told them they had to push aside *their* barriers, just as the readers need to. We all need to allow ourselves the opportunity to not only think of end of life planning, but to think of it in a different way.

"End of life planning isn't fatal. End of life planning is preparation."

They said to me, "but it's not a very upbeat subject." I smiled at them and replied that I believe just the opposite. End of life planning is the witnessing of one's whole life: piece by piece, accomplishment by accomplishment, your life puzzle is assembled—and that includes making sure the last few pieces are in place. Not only is this a powerful experience personally, but I know from experience that when I talked about these issues with my family, our bonds became tighter and stronger.

Here's the thing, dear Reader: we rarely take the time to contemplate life. Let me say that again, because it's easy to miss that powerful little sentence: We rarely take the time to contemplate life. Why? Because there's so darn much going on that we can hardly see the life itself. But when you sit down in your quiet place—let's say in a favorite chair—and turn off the distractions, and think about your great journey and your end of life plan, it can be joyful. It can be liberating. It can be uplifting.

End of life planning isn't fatal. End of life planning is preparation. It can and should be done well in advance of death. In my case, when I settled into my favorite chair and let the late-night quiet wrap around me, I looked at the smiling faces on family pictures surrounding me. I allowed myself to celebrate those captured moments and the many milestones that brought me to this moment.

As I sunk deeper into my chair, I gave myself the space to sink deeper into thought. My mind was at peace, enough so that I could contemplate the arc of life—the good fortunes and the bad—and the many accomplishments I've been blessed with. More so, I thought about the glorious days ahead.

This moment of quiet opened doors for me, and you should let it do the same for you. These doors had been shut and locked by endless to-do lists and schedules and worries, but the peace and quiet unlocked them. By making time for quiet thought, I was able to rededicate myself to all the things that I still want to do in life. It allowed me think about the relationships I have with the people I love and who love me. It helped me solidify those relationships and indulge myself in that love. It reminded me that for their sake, as well as mine, I wanted to be more attentive to my health, now and as I continue to age.

In this chapter, we will discuss the different elements of end of life planning. We'll talk about your advance directive (often called a living will), and your decision on where you'd prefer to be when your life ends: most commonly, your options include home, a hospice facility, a nursing home, or a hospital. We'll also discuss the important decision of organ donation.

> **END OF LIFE PLANNING**
>
> - Complete and discuss your advance directive
> - Communicate your wishes on where you would prefer to die
> - Communicate your wishes on organ donation

As a country, we need to rethink how we deal with end of life planning. This subject shouldn't be something we approach with fear. It shouldn't be taboo. It should be done in the full light of a life well lived. Think of this as your opportunity to celebrate your complete life puzzle. End of life planning is knowing the satisfaction of snapping in those last few pieces.

My appeal to you: push away the distractions and the barriers keeping you from such thoughts. Find a comfortable space and some quiet time. Start to formulate your plan. Rather than considering end of life planning as a downer, think of it as uplifting. A great sense of accomplishment, peace, and control will come over you as you embrace this process. Take charge. Control what you can control. Enjoy the discovery that comes with contemplating one's purpose in life. There is peace in reflecting on the many accomplishments behind you. And there is joy in striving for the many goals still ahead.

> **"An advance directive ensures the preservation of your personal dignity and integrity as a human being."**

✚ WHAT IS AN ADVANCE DIRECTIVE?

An advance directive is a legal document that allows you to express your wishes concerning medical decisions and treatment at the end life. It also identifies who will speak for you if you can no longer take charge of your health care decisions.

But that's the technical definition.

Said another way, an advance directive is one of the truest examples of taking control of your life, and telling your family and the medical system how you want to be cared for at the end of your life. It ensures the preservation of your autonomy and personal dignity and integrity as a human being. This document contains your clear instructions on what you do and do not want done regarding life-sustaining treatments and other medical decisions.

In general, an advance directive consists of two parts. First, a living will, which states your wishes, among other things, regarding the use or nonuse of life support interventions. Second, your advance directive will designate health care power of

DR. YOU MEDICAL NOTE:

Fewer than 50% of severely or terminally ill seniors have completed an advance directive.

attorney to someone who you trust to speak on behalf of your wishes. This person is called your health advocate, health surrogate, or health proxy, depending on what state you live in.

The fact is, we all need to plan before crisis arrives. An advance directive causes us to take, arguably, the most significant look in the mirror that Dr. You will encounter. This is you taking charge. This is you saying, "Here is how I want the end of my life handled." An advance directive is Dr. You's final orders, and among the most important ones you'll ever hand out. This document is legally binding under (and only under) the following stipulations:

- Two physicians have certified that you are unable to make medical decisions for yourself.

- You are in a medical condition specified in the state's living will law, such as "terminal illness" or "permanent unconsciousness."

- Other requirements may apply, depending on state law.

It's imperative that you share your advance directive decisions with family, but ultimately, these are your decisions to make. If you have questions or would appreciate advice and discussion from your physician, attorney, clergy, or loved ones while completing the document, that's perfectly normal. There is no one "right way" to fill out an advance directive. Ultimately, you need to make these decisions from the heart. No one has access to the guidance of your heart but you.

"You have to get over any fears you might have of an advance directive, and then help your family get over theirs."

As you fill out your advance directive, you need to make a very important decision: whom do you trust to speak on your behalf, to see to it that your wishes are carried out? Without an advance directive specifying your health advocate, the state will choose your advocate on your behalf. This is not the best way forward—since when does the state know you well enough to make such a personal decision for you?

You'd be amazed by all the people that I speak with who don't have advance directives. The latest statistic I saw said fewer than 50% of severely or terminally ill seniors have completed one.[1] That means the chances of medical treatment at the end of life being carried out specifically to someone's wishes are about as good as a coin flip. How wrong is that?

What's keeping people from filling out an advance directive? Well, as we talked about already: things like fear and the constant press of life's daily responsibilities are barriers. What I also see is a situation where everyone is waiting for someone else to start the conversation. Patients, many times, believe that their physician should start the conversation. Adult children think their parents should initiate the discussion. Everyone is waiting for the other, like some never-ending staredown. It's a stalemate of silence.

"An advance directive is the gift of clarity. Gifts and celebrations go together, right?"

Let me break the silence: start the conversation! You may want to do so with your advance directive in hand, in which case you're discussing the decisions that you've reflected upon already. Or you can use the conversation as a starting point to fill out your advance directive. There's no one correct way other than to do what feels right for you. And while you're at it, encourage friends and family to get going on their advance directives, too.

Advance directives do vary from state to state, so be sure to fill out yours in accordance with your state's laws. The two sources I suggest for more complete information on advance directives are: Aging with Dignity at www.agingwithdignity. org; look for Five Wishes (also be sure to look at Five Wishes Online). The other tremendous resource is Caring Connections at www.caringinfo.org. You'll find everything you need there. We're lucky to have sources like this to consult.

✚ LET YOUR FAMILY KNOW YOUR WISHES

After I discussed my advance directive with my wife and physician—and then completed the document—do you know what? I felt really, really good. A burden was lifted. My plan was in place. It was similar to the feeling I used to get in med school when all my homework was done. I knew I was prepared, and the worry vanished.

Now it was time to involve my family. The whole family. I'm telling you, even if you have an eccentric sister who lives in a mountain shack and survives on organic vegetables and rainwater, you need to involve her, too. Otherwise she could claim—rather forcefully—that she knows your wishes when she doesn't.

Communicate your end of life wishes clearly to the entire family, or to a good friend if that is the person who will be acting on your behalf. Remember to designate one health advocate or health surrogate from your family or group of friends. It's their responsibility to speak for you to ensure that your wishes are upheld. End of life care can be nuanced and complex; a candid conversation helps you transfer your written wishes and your deeper philosophy on these issues to loved ones.

Many of us worry that if we have this discussion—especially with our children—it might upset them. There might even be tears shed. None of us want to see our children upset,

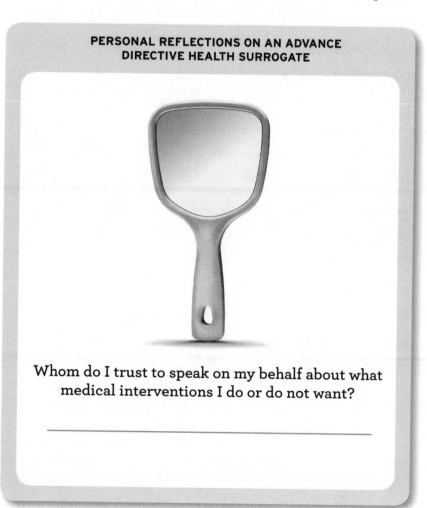

PERSONAL REFLECTIONS ON AN ADVANCE DIRECTIVE HEALTH SURROGATE

Whom do I trust to speak on my behalf about what medical interventions I do or do not want?

_____

but we can't let this become an excuse. You may need to explain to your family, as I explained to you earlier in this section, that end of life planning is nothing to be afraid of. Tell them that filling out an advance directive gave you a rare chance to sit down, clear some mental space, and contemplate life's many gifts. Tell them it also offered you the opportunity to look forward, to aspirations and dreams ahead. This should break the ice, so to speak, let everyone take a deep breath, and create room for the conversation to flourish.

Where do you do this? How do you do this? There are as many different ways to share your advance directive with family as there are different families. Just go back to our key point: this doesn't have to be a somber occasion. Quite the contrary! This is a chance to bring the family together and share in your love. In my case, we had a party. And perhaps so should you.

✚ REASON TO CELEBRATE?

When I talked to my family about my advance directive, I started by reminding them that just like with other end of life planning decisions, filling out this document is not fatal, nor should it be perceived as an admission of any kind. It's simply one of the natural steps in healthy aging.

See that word "advance" preceding the word "directive"? This means that you are thinking in advance—isn't that what wise and prudent people do? That certainly is what a well-informed Dr. You does. An advance directive is the gift of clarity. Gifts and celebrations go together, right? So why not celebrate? Take away the fear. Get everyone thinking about this subject in a new, positive light.

Some of the best times to get together for an advance directive party are the holidays like Thanksgiving or Christmas when family naturally gathers. If you can't get your hyper-busy twenty-first century family together in person, wrangle them using that twenty-first century invention called a smartphone. That's right. Put together a conference call. If you don't know how, have one of your hyper-busy twenty-first century sons or daughters facilitate it. If all else fails, Google "conference call [your phone model]" to find out how it's done. As you can see, I'm serious about you doing this. There's no excuse not to.

If you're still having trouble finding the right occasion to have these end of life discussions, here's a no-fail idea. Use April 16 as your springboard to get the conversation and the party started. Every year since 2008, the country has used April 16 to celebrate National Healthcare Decision Day, a nationwide program to help provide information and get the conversation started on advance directives and more. You can find additional information at www.nhdd.org. So if you're stuck, tell yourself and your family, April 16 is the day.

✚ IS ALL OF THIS REALLY NECESSARY?

Contemplating end of life medical decisions requires some serious thought, and the research I've seen shows it's darn well worth it. Do you think your spouse knows your end of life wishes? How about your doctor? Surely your doctor knows, right? If you said yes, think again.

I have seen studies where spouses or partners have been separated and put into different rooms. Each was asked about the other's wishes for medical treatment at the end of life. Guess what? Most often, the separated couple didn't know each other's wishes.

"The focus of hospice is on caring, not curing."

Next, doctors and their patients were separated. They were asked about end of life preferences. And again, they weren't on the same page. Why? Two primary reasons. First, we are not a death-defying culture, we are a death-denying culture. As a general rule, we just don't talk about this stuff. Second, we're not on the same page because there is no page. People need a process and structure for sitting down and getting their wishes on paper. Otherwise the mere thought of it can be overwhelming.

This is your time to prevent things you don't want to happen, and ensure what does happen is in accordance with your wishes. You are in charge of telling the doctors and hospitals want you want. You are in charge of telling your family what you want. So tell them. That's what they've been waiting to hear. As it turns out, it's a big relief for all involved.

End of life can be traumatic. Oftentimes, people aren't thinking clearly. An advance directive brings clarity to the room. It lets you focus on a loved one's life rather than argue about a loved one's death. Isn't that the way it should be?

✚ OTHER ADVANCE DIRECTIVE CONSIDERATIONS

You should be aware that emergency medical technicians and other first responders cannot honor living wills or medical powers of attorney. Upon arriving at a home, an accident site, or a care facility, they are required to do everything necessary to stabilize a person for transfer to a hospital.

There are additional documents and forms called DNR (do not resuscitate), or in some states, DNAR (do not attempt resuscitation), or AND (allow natural death). Another more comprehensive order is POLST (physician's orders for life-sustaining treatment), or in some states, MOLST (medical orders for life-sustaining treatment), that you and your physician fill out, and your physician signs. These documents are intended for those who are seriously ill and want their wishes

DR. YOU MEDICAL NOTE:

90% of people say that they want to die at home. Yet nearly 80% of people die in institutions like a hospital or nursing home.

for life-sustaining treatments honored across all health care settings. They function as medical orders from your doctor that direct first responders at the scene of an emergency. For more information, talk to your health care team.

A few final thoughts. Your advance directive is legally valid in the United States, but the laws governing it oftentimes vary from state to state. Be sure that the advance directive that you fill out and sign is in compliance with your state's laws.

You do not need a lawyer to fill out your document, but be sure to sign it in front of the required witnesses (in some cases notarization is required).

Advance directives do not expire. They can and should be updated as your health status and wishes change. Again, see these two sources for more detailed information: Aging with Dignity at www.agingwithdignity.org, and Caring Connections at www.caringinfo.org.

Lastly, make sure that your advance directive is accessible. One copy should go to your health care power of attorney, and another to your primary care physician. I also suggest you store your document electronically (yes, it will be safe and secure) at the U.S. Living Will Registry®. See www.livingwillregistry.com for simple guidance.

✚ DEFINE QUALITY OF LIFE FOR YOU

Many end of life planning decisions commonly revolve around quality of life issues. How much pain is too much pain? How much suffering is too much suffering?

Too often family members and your medical team have to guess at these elusive measures. That's an impossible task. For some, quality of life means being mentally alert, flashing an occasional twinkle in the eye, and not depending on a feeding tube for nutrition. For others, it's feeling the sunshine on their face. And for others still, there is quality in life no matter what, and all means medically possible should be employed to extend it.

Quality of life has physical, emotional, and spiritual considerations. You need to tell your family and medical team what constitutes quality of life for you, and when that quality is no longer present, what measures—if any—you want taken.

For one woman who had terminal cancer, her quality of life meant holding fast to the idea of seeing her young child walk down the aisle on his wedding day. When it became clear that nothing could be medically done to extend her life that length of time, she did the next best thing. She videotaped the speech she wanted him to hear at his wedding reception. The tape

DR. YOU MEDICAL NOTE:

For more on hospice care, go to the National Hospice and Palliative Care Organization (NHPCO) at www.caringinfo.org. Or call the NHPCO Helpline at 800-658-8898.

was put aside in the boy's safety deposit box. She will be there when her little boy strides into adulthood as a new groom. The woman passed away peacefully less than a week after finishing her gift to her son.

Your goals and wishes for medical care during end of life are so personal that they have to be documented to be properly honored. Many times such wishes include your choice on where you would prefer to die, and the care that you wish to receive there. For many that choice includes hospice care. It's a beautiful way to celebrate a life, surrounded by family and dear friends, when the end is near.

✚ HOSPICE

Where's the best place to die? Only you can answer this for yourself. When The Gallup Organization posed this question to people, 90% of respondents said they wanted to die at home. Yet currently, nearly 80% of people die in institutions like a hospital or nursing home. As you can see, wishes and reality are not in alignment.

As I see it, based on the many people I talk to, part of the reason for this disconnect is that people don't realize the level and quality of care that can be provided to the terminally ill at home. If your family is there to support your wishes, in most situations, hospice care can be given at home.

You see, hospice isn't a *place*; hospice is comfort, support, and care for a person at the end of life. Hospice care also includes support for family members and friends. Beyond being provided at home, hospice care can be received in a home-like setting at an inpatient facility. The decision about where to receive hospice has much to do with the patient's wishes and capabilities of the family.

Hospice can be received when two physicians conclude that if a serious illness takes its natural course, death within six months would not be a surprise. The focus of hospice is on caring, not curing. It's a team approach to end of life, including a doctor, nurse, social worker, counselor, chaplain, home health aide, and trained volunteers. The emphasis is on managing pain and other symptoms, while being sensitive to the special requirements of the family. Some people I talk to think hospice hastens death. That is a myth. Hospice neither hastens nor postpones death.

Medicare, Medicaid, private insurance plans, HMOs, and other managed care organizations almost always provide hospice benefits. There are many factors that go into selecting the

DR. YOU MEDICAL NOTE:

Medicare, Medicaid, private insurance plans, HMOs, and other managed care organizations almost always provide hospice benefits.

right hospice program. You'll want to ask questions about things like certification, federal oversight, if clinical and other staff are available 24/7, and how long the program has been in the community, to name a few. For a complete list of questions to help you manage this process, and more information, go to the National Hospice and Palliative Care Organization (NHPCO) at www.caringinfo.org where you can click on Choosing a Hospice for a printable worksheet. Or call the NHPCO Helpline at 800-658-8898.

As I said before, these are deeply personal decisions, but as a professional who has spent his whole life in medical care, I will tell you that hospice at home or in a facility is very often a better place to say goodbye to a loved one than a hospital, with its limited visiting hours and impersonal surroundings. And most hospital health professionals will tell you the same thing.

I urge you to discuss the possibility of hospice with your family. If hospice is something you want as part of your end of life plan, please remember to document that in your advance directive.

✚ THE GREATEST GIFT: BE AN ORGAN DONOR

I want to tell you about my amazing son, Kobie. Kobie passed away not long ago. It's unspeakably tragic to lose a young son, but I'm so proud of him. Kobie had made the decision to be an organ donor. Because of that unselfish act, a man who works as an elementary school aide has Kobie's heart. He is married and has two children. Another man, a retired truck driver and father of four, was gifted Kobie's lungs. Thanks to Kobie, he is still pursuing his hobbies of playing guitar, gardening, and fishing. And yet another man, this one a young student who had been on a waiting list for two years, was gifted Kobie's kidney. He, and many others, have had their dreams for a new life realized because of Kobie's generosity.

It is so important that you too become an organ donor. And not just you—be sure to talk to your children and grandchildren about the remarkable gift they can offer to others.

My Kobie is a miracle in my life. And Kobie, by way of organ donation, is now a miracle for others, and for their children and families. I'm so proud that my son lives on.

Did you know that anyone, regardless of age or medical history, can register to be an organ donor? What's more, did you know it's a fact that most religions in the U.S. support organ donation and consider this gift a final act of love and generosity toward your fellow man?

In less time than it takes to read this chapter—every 11 minutes—another person is added to the organ donor list. The need is great, but so too is the generosity of people like Kobie, and like you.

One day I was giving a healthy aging presentation to a large group of 50-somethings—a presentation, by the way, that became the genesis for this book. In my presentation, I had shared my story about Kobie and his gifts to others. Afterward, a woman approached me and shared a story that I will never forget. It was the story of another woman who, like me, had lost her young African-American son, who was also an organ donor. A few years after her loss, this woman decided to seek out the recipients of her beloved son's organs. She wanted to see what miracles they were working.

Her journey took her to the South. Across freeways, through winding county highways, and finally, down a rut-ted road in rural Appalachia. She knocked on a screened door whose address matched the one she held on a folded piece of paper. When the door opened, she stood face-to-face with a man who looked as different from her as humanly possible. The burly man was as tall as the doorframe, his white skin tanned from years of hard work outdoors. They looked at one another, their eyes searching for some explanation. Finally, gracefully, he stepped toward her, and carefully embraced her, and gently took her head and put it to his chest. In a thick mountain accent, the man said, "Listen to your son."

"Please consider the gift of organ donation, and ask your family to do so, too."

What a gift organ donation is. It is the perfect living example of how we are all vulnerable, how we are all interconnected, and how we all are in need of one another's profoundly unselfish acts. Please, go to donatelife.net and learn more about organ donation. And encourage those you love to do so as well.

✛ I HOPE TO SEE YOU DOWN THE ROAD

Dear Reader, our time together is coming to a close—but just for the moment. Let me say what a pleasure it's been meeting you through these pages and how lucky I am to be able to share my passion for healthy living with you.

I'm so proud to be your partner in health. You've gone to the mirror and had an honest look at your strengths and weaknesses. You've taken your health in your own hands and done the very best you can to prevent disease. You've looked at your lifestyle and added a bit more exercise and social activity to it.

You've started to eat a healthier diet by paying greater attention to what goes in your grocery cart and on your plate. You better understand your medicine, and the goals for each and every medication. You've picked the right doctor and the right hospital and the right health plan. You've improved the health and safety of your home and woven your safety net. Your end of life plans are in place. Sit back for a moment and relish it. If you still have a ways to go, don't be discouraged. Be determined. You can do it. Remember, the secret is a penny at a time.

"If you'd like to talk more about your health, share a success story, or a struggle, drop me a line at www.doctorinthemirror.com."

Dr. You, it's been my distinct pleasure. Hopefully, in my travels, we'll meet again. Perhaps I'll be in an airport, or sitting at a coffee shop, or giving a commencement address at your grandchild's graduation, and you'll come over. I'll know who you are. I'll recognize you right off as someone who is doing their best to control what they can control and age with health, joy, and vitality.

I truly believe this conversation is just a beginning, more than it is something coming to an end. I'll see you down the road, and we can pick up where we left off. In the meantime, if you'd like to talk more about your health, share a success story, or a struggle, drop me a line at www.doctorinthemirror.com.

Take care of yourself, dear Reader. You're worth it. You are so worth it.

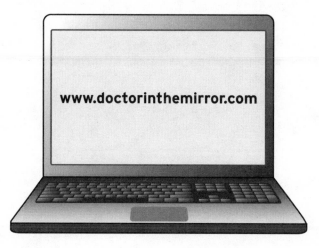

DOCTOR'S ORDERS
END OF LIFE PLANNING

℞

- Don't think of end of life planning as somber or frightening. It's a celebration of the life you've lived, and the life ahead of you.

- End of life planning requires completing your advance directive, discussing wishes about where you'd prefer to die, and your wishes for organ donation.

- Fill out your advance directive. It's one of the truest examples of taking control of your life, and telling your family and the medical system how you want your life to end.

- Designate one health advocate or health surrogate from your family or group of friends.

- Bring your family and loved ones together and celebrate your life by discussing your advance directive.

- Define what "quality of life" is for you so your family and medical team know what measures— if any—you want taken should that quality be impaired.

- Find out about hospice care. If it's your preference for end of life, discuss it and document it.

- Please consider the gift of organ donation, and ask your family to do so, too.

Dr. You

W E B S I T E S

CHAPTER 1: HEALTH IN AMERICA
Skin cancer: www.cdc.gov/cancer/skin/basic_info/prevention.html
Exercise: www.easyforyou.info
Alzheimer's: www.alz.org
Alzheimer's: www.nia.nih.gov/alzheimers
Depression: www.nimh.nih.gov
Incontinence: www.nia.nih.gov/HealthInformation/Publications/
urinary.html
Anemia: www.healthinaging.org
Arthritis: www.arthritis.org

CHAPTER 2: BAD HABITS
Worker safety: www.osha.gov
Body mass index: www.nhlbisupport.com/bmi/
Obesity: www.thiscityisgoingonadiet.com

CHAPTER 3: HEALTHY DIET
Healthy eating: www.choosemyplate.gov
Calorie calculator: www.mayoclinic.com/health/calorie-calculator/
NU00598

CHAPTER 4: BE ACTIVE
Exercise: www.easyforyou.info
Exercise: www.nia.nih.gov/HealthInformation/Publications/Exer-
ciseGuide/
Exercise: www.eldergym.com
Battling obesity: www.thiscityisgoingonadiet.com

CHAPTER 5: DOCTOR VISITS
Physician quality: www.careaboutyourcare.org
Physician quality: www.ncqa.org
Physician quality: www.docboard.org
Free eye exam: www.eyecareamerica.org

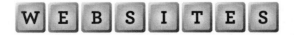

CHAPTER 6: PRESCRIPTION DRUGS AND MEDICATIONS
Drug interactions: www.drugdigest.org

CHAPTER 7: HOSPITALIZATION
Hospital quality: www.ahrq.gov
Hospital quality: www.hospitalcompare.hhs.gov
Hospital quality: www.leapfroggroup.org
In-home heath care: www.aoa.gov
In-home health care: www.eldercare.gov

CHAPTER 8: THE RIGHT HEALTH INSURANCE PLAN
Health insurance basics: www.medicare.gov
Benefit eligibility: www.benefits.gov
State assistance: www.shiptalk.org

CHAPTER 10: CREATING YOUR PERSONAL SAFETY NET
Caregiving tips: www.aarp.org
Caregiving tips: www.caregiver.org
Caregiving tips: www.caregiving.org
Caregiving tips: www.fullcirclecare.org
Elder abuse: www.apsnetwork.org
Elder abuse: www.ncea.aoa.gov
In-home care: www.services4aging.org
Caregiving resources: www.care.com
Senior services: www.seniorslist.com
Shared living: www.nationalsharedhousing.org
Nursing homes: www.medicare.gov/NHCompare

CHAPTER 11: END OF LIFE PLANNING
Advance directive: www.agingwithdignity.org
Advance directive: www.caringinfo.org
Advance directive: www.nhdd.org
Dr. Reed's website: www.doctorinthemirror.com

ENDNOTES

CHAPTER 1

[1]   Source: Central Intelligence Agency
https://www.cia.gov/library/publications/the-world-factbook/
rankorder/2102rank.html

[2]   Source: Neonatal Mortality Levels for 193 Countries in 2009 with
Trends since 1990: A Systematic Analysis of Progress,
Projections, and Priorities
PLoS Medicine, August 2011

[3]   Source: United Nations Statistical Division, updated June 2011 http://
unstats.un.org/unsd/demographic/products/socind/health.htm

[4]   Office of the Actuary, Centers for Medicare & Medicaid

[5]   Office of the Actuary, Centers for Medicare & Medicaid

[6]   Source: STATEMENT OF KEN DYCHTWALD, PRESIDENT AND
CHIEF EXECUTIVE OFFICER, AGE WAVE, SAN FRANCISCO,
CA at U.S. Senate Hearing "BREAKING THE SILVER CEILING: A
NEW GENERATION OF OLDER AMERICANS REDEFINING
THE NEW RULES OF THE WORKPLACE," September 20, 2004
http://ftp.resource.org/gpo.gov/hearings/108s/97086.txt

[7]   U.S. National Institute of Health

[8]   "Health-Related Quality of Life of U.S. Adults with Arthritis: Analysis
of Data from the Behavioral Risk Factor Surveillance System, 2003, 2005,
and 2007." Sylvia E. Furner, Jennifer M. Hootman, Charles G. Helmick,
Julie Bolen, Matthew M. Zack. Arthritis Care and Research; Published
Online: April 28, 2011 (DOI: 10.1002/acr.20430). http://doi.wiley.
com/10.1002/acr.20430

[9]   Source: National Vital Statistics Reports, Vol 59, No 4, CDC, March 16,
2011 http://www.cdc.gov/nchs/data/nvsr/nvsr59/nvsr59_04.pdf

[10]   Source: Cancer Facts & Figures 2011 – American Cancer Society
         http://www.cancer.org/acs/groups/content/@epidemiologysurveilance/
         documents/document/acspc-029771.pdf

[11]   Source: Alzheimer's Facts & Figures 2010, Alzheimer's Association
         http://www.alz.org/documents_custom/report_alzfactsfigures2010.pdf

[12]   Source: Death in the United States, 2009, CDC NCHS Data Brief • No.
         64 • July 2011 http://www.cdc.gov/nchs/data/databriefs/db64.pdf

[13]   Levy BR, et al. Longevity increased by positive self-perceptions of aging.
         Journal of Personality and Social Psychology. 2002 Aug; 83(2):261-70.
         http://www.apa.org/pubs/journals/releases/psp-832261.pdf

[14]   Source: White House Budget FY 2010 http://www.whitehouse.gov/sites/
         default/files/omb/budget/fy2012/assets/tables.pdf

[15]   Source: Projections of Education Statistics to 2019, Nation Center for
         Education Statistics, US Department of Education, 2011 http://nces.
         ed.gov/pubs2011/2011017.pdf

[16]   Source: Morbidity and Mortality Weekly Report, Center for Disease
         Control & Prevention, November 13, 2008 http://www.cdc.gov/mmwr/
         PDF/wk/mm5745.pdf

[17]   Source: The Future Costs of Obesity: National and State Estimates of
         the Impact of Obesity on Direct Health Care Expenses, United Health
         Foundation, the American Public Health Association and Partnership for
         Prevention, November 2009 http://www.fightchronicdisease.org/sites/

         default/files/docs/CostofObesityReport-FINAL.pdf

CHAPTER 2

[1]   Source: Behavior Matters, American Journal of Prevention, 2011

[2/3]   Source: Cancer Facts & Figures 2011 – American Cancer Society
         http://www.cancer.org/acs/groups/content/@epidemiologysurveilance/
         documents/document/acspc-029771.pdf

[4]   Source: Cancer Facts & Figures, 2001—American Cancer Society

[5]   Source: Youth & Tobacco Use, CDC accessed August 2, 2011 http://
         www.cdc.gov/tobacco/data_statistics/fact_sheets/youth_data/tobacco_use/
         index.htm

[6]   Source: Cancer Facts & Figures 2011 – American Cancer Society
        http://www.cancer.org/acs/groups/content/@epidemiologysurveilance/
        documents/document/acspc-029771.pdf

[7]   Source: Cancer Facts & Figures 2011 – American Cancer Society
        http://www.cancer.org/acs/groups/content/@epidemiologysurveilance/
        documents/document/acspc-029771.pdf

[8]   Source: Cancer Facts & Figures 2011 – American Cancer Society
        http://www.cancer.org/acs/groups/content/@epidemiologysurveilance/
        documents/document/acspc-029771.pdf

[9]   Source: University of Minnesota research as cited in "Obese shrug off risk
        to health," Pioneer Press, December 2, 2010, by Christopher Snowbeck,

[10]   Reference: Christakis, N.A., and Fowler, J.H. The spread of obesity in
        a large social network over 32 years. New England Journal of Medicine
        (2007), 357(4):370-379. http://christakis.med.harvard.edu/pdf/

        publications/articles/078.pdf

[11]   Source: Nielson Company

[12]   Source: Nielson Company

[13]   Department of Exercise Science, Arnold School of Public Health,
        University of South Carolina, Columbia, SC 29208, USA. warrenty
        mailbox.sc.edu http://www.ncbi.nlm.nih.gov/pubmed/19996993

CHAPTER 3

[1]   Source: Int J Behav Nutr Phys Act. 2008; 5: 9.
        Published online 2008 February 12. doi: 10.1186/1479-5868-5-9
        http://www.ncbi.nlm.nih.gov/pmc/articles/PMC2275297/

[2]   Source: Health, United States, 2010, CDC, http://www.cdc.gov/nchs/
        data/hus/hus10.pdf

[3]   Source: FDA plans to limit amount of salt allowed in processed
        foods for health reasons, Washington Post, April 20, 2010 http://
        www.washingtonpost.com/wp-dyn/content/article/2010/04/19/
        AR2010041905049.html

[4]   Source: Strategies to Reduce Sodium Intake in the United States,
        Institute of Medicine, April 2010

[5]   Source: CLINICAL GUIDELINES ON THE IDENTIFICATION, EVALUATION, AND TREATMENT OF OVERWEIGHT AND OBESITY IN ADULTS, National Institutes of Health http://www.nhlbi.nih.gov/guidelines/obesity/ob_gdlns.pdf

CHAPTER 4

[1]   Source: http://www.infoplease.com/dk/science/encyclopedia/muscular-system.html

[2]   Source: Sarcopenia, long term care and nutritional implications, conference presentation by Nutricia Advanced Medical Nutrition-Paul Rigby, December 2, 2010

[3]   Source: 2008 National Population Projections, US Census Bureau http://www.census.gov/population/www/projections/2008projections.html

[4]   Source: Big-spending Boomers bend rules of marketing, USA Today, December 15, 2010 http://www.usatoday.com/money/advertising/2010-11-15-babyboomers-spending_N.htm

[5]   Source: US Census, Reported Rates of Voting and Registration by Selected Characteristics: 2008, http://www.census.gov/prod/2010pubs/p20-562.pdf

[6]   Source: A Clear Rejection of the Status Quo, No Consensus about Future Policies, Pew Research, November 3, 2010 updated November 17, 2010 http://pewresearch.org/pubs/1789/2010-midterm-elections-exit-poll-analysis

[7]   Source: SEXUAL HEALTH AN ISSUE FOR BOOMERS, The Baltimore Sun, June 2, 2011, by Marni Jameson

CHAPTER 5

[1]   Source: Adult Immunization: Shots to Save Lives, Robert Wood Johnson Foundation & Trust for America's Health, February 2010 http://healthyamericans.org/assets/files/TFAH2010AdultImmnzBrief13.pdf

[2]   Source: Influenza Vaccination of Adults, CDC - National Center for Immunization and Respiratory Diseases, Carolyn B. Bridges, MD - Associate Director for Science, Influenza Division, December 9, 2010 www.cdc.gov/vaccines/ed/ciinc/downloads/Dec_10/Bridges.pptx

[3]   Source: Health Interview Survey – Receipt of Influenza
        Vaccination, CDC, June 2011 http://www.cdc.gov/nchs/data/nhis/
        earlyrelease/201106_04.pdf

[4]   Source: National Vital Statistics Reports, Vol 59, No 4, CDC, March 16,
        2011 http://www.cdc.gov/nchs/data/nvsr/nvsr59/nvsr59_04.pdf

CHAPTER 6

[1]   Prescription Drug Use Continues to Increase: U.S. Prescription Drug Data
        2007-2008, NCHS Data Brief No. 42, September 2010

[2]   Source: Prescription Drug Trends, Kaiser Family Foundation, http://www.
        kff.org/rxdrugs/upload/3057-08.pdf

[3]   Manasse HR. (1989). Medication use in an imperfect world: Drug
        misadventuring as an issue of public policy. Part 1. Am J Hosp Pharm, 46:
        929–944.

CHAPTER 7

[1]   Source: "How to Avoid the Round-Trip Visit to the Hospital," Navigating
        the Health Care System
        Advice Columns from Dr. Carolyn Clancy, AHRQ, June 1, 2010
        http://www.ahrq.gov/consumer/cc/cc060110.htm

[2]   Source: A Healthier Life? It's Up To You! UnitedHealth Group, Orlando
        @ 50+, page 42

[3]   Source: Statistical Brief # 94 - Adult Hospital Stays with Infections Due
        to Medical Care, 2007, HCUP-Agency for Healthcare Research and
        Quality, August 2010 http://www.hcup-us.ahrq.gov/reports/statbriefs/
        sb94.jsp

[4]   Source: ADVERSE EVENTS IN HOSPITALS: NATIONAL
        INCIDENCE AMONG MEDICARE BENEFICIARIES, US Dept of
        Health and Human Services - Office of the Inspector General, November
        2010 http://oig.hhs.gov/oei/reports/oei-06-09-00090.pdf

CHAPTER 9

[1]   Source: US Department of Health and Human Services – Administration on Aging, Health, Prevention and Wellness Program http://www.aoa.gov/AoARoot/AoA_Programs/HCLTC/Evidence_Based/index.aspx

[2]   UnitedHealthcare in consultation with AARP Services, Inc "Falls and Risk of Falling Have Greater Impact on Older Adults' Quality of Life Than Diabetes, Hypertension and Other Chronic Conditions.

[3]   Source: Centers for Disease Control   http://www.cdc.gov/HomeandRecreationalSafety/Falls/adulthipfx.html

[4]   Source: Vital Signs-May 2011, CDC http://www.cdc.gov/VitalSigns/Asthma/index.html

CHAPTER 10

[1]   Source: The MetLife Study of Caregiving Costs to Working Caregivers, MetLife Mature Market Institute, June 2011 http://www.caregiving.org/wp-content/uploads/2011/06/mmi-caregiving-costs-working-caregivers.pdf

[2]   Source: Caregiving in the U.S. 2009, National Alliance for Caregiving in collaboration with AARP, November 2009 http://www.caregiving.org/data/Caregiving_in_the_US_2009_full_report.pdf

CHAPTER 11

[1]   (U.S. Agency for Healthcare Research Quality 2003 "Advance Care Planning: Preferences for Care at the end of life) http://www.ahrq.gov/research/endliferia/endria.pdf

INDEX

Z